VENERATING THE ROOT

VENERATING THE ROOT

Sūn Sīmiǎo's
Bèi Jí Qiān Jīn Yào Fāng

(Essential Prescriptions Worth a Thousand in
Gold for Every Emergency)

孫思邈

備急千金要方

Volume 5: Pediatrics

卷五：少小嬰孺方

Translated by Sabine Wilms

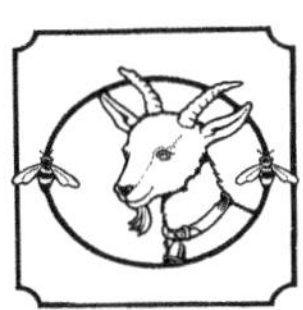

HAPPY GOAT PRODUCTIONS

CORBETT, OREGON

Published by Happy Goat Productions
Corbett, OR

Venerating the Root, Part 1: A Translation of Sūn Sīmiǎo's Volume on Pediatrics in the Bèi Jí Qiān Jīn Yào Fāng; translation and commmentary by Sabine Wilms

Printed in the United States of America

ISBN-978-0-9913429-0-7

Book design and layout by Kimberly Gray
Cover art by Sunjae Lee

This book is dedicated to my root, my grandmother Ellinor Wilms, proud pediatrician and lover of children and beauty and music, and to my fruit, my daughter Momo. And to all mothers and fathers and gentle souls who cover children's ears during thunderstorms.

Contents

Foreword

Sūn Sīmiǎo understood the importance of treating children, of setting up a strong constitution for a healthy life ahead. He also writes of not treating, of understanding and respecting the body's own wisdom to clear and cleanse through its own unfolding processes, such as in the early childhood cycles of transformation and steaming, *bian zheng*. This refreshing respect for the innate intelligence of emerging life, his constant attention to detail in signs and symptoms, diagnostics, treatment strategies and health advice, his interest in the personality of the child and indications for longevity, his care to protect and at the same time not over-protect, and his awareness of the all too real possibility of harm from crude and inappropriate treatments, all these are aspects we can learn from today. I hope that Sabine's great work to make Sūn Sīmiǎo's perspective and teaching accessible to all will encourage and stimulate practitioners to deepen their own practice of pediatrics. For a healthy future, there can be no more important study.

Peter Firebrace
8th December 2013

Another treasure of Chinese medicine literature has been unearthed and made available to the Western student. In reading Sūn Sīmiǎo's medical encyclopedia it is easy to see why he is considered through the ages as one of the most illuminated minds of Chinese medicine, even ascending to the status of demigod or immortal in popular lore. Not only did Sūn Sīmiǎo systematically record any and all medical knowledge known to him to have clinical relevance, laboriously copying many of the Classics that preceded him as well as recipes used by different lineages and practitioners of his time, but he also in many cases elucidates the mysteries therein by offering commentaries or explanations of theories and formulae.

Reading Sūn Sīmiǎo's *Bèi Jí Qiān Jīn Yào Fāng* my impression is that of a comprehensive resource, one that provides access to canonical classical texts and to many formulae elaborated from the understanding of these theories, as well as to the voice of old master Sūn making sure the student of Chinese medicine understands the subtleties of certain patterns and presentations. He leads our way, taking great care to compare signs and symptoms, formulae and single ingredients, always emphasizing where one might make a mistake and pointing the way to ascertain correct diagnosis. This makes the *Bèi Jí Qiān Jīn Yào Fāng* a priceless resource for any student/practitioner, especially in this modern age where much of classical Chinese medicine has been lost or diluted by the history of the 20th century.

Indeed modern western Chinese medicine schools barely teach the Classics, and rarely teach pediatrics. These two aspects of our medicine are therefore not easily accessible to the majority of western students. This present volume on "Nurturing the Root" fills a great part of this significant gap in our education: it presents a comprehensive overview of neonatal and pediatric classical physiology, neonatal care including cord care, grooming and breastfeeding, and diseases that are proper to children. The first pearl of wisdom from Master Sūn is in informing us that most pediatric diseases are the same as adult ones, and should be treated according to the same governing principles - except for the ones he delineates in this volume.

Sūn Sīmiǎo begins by describing normal neonatal physiology, describing the phases of development from birth to the early years. Such physiological theory is absolutely fundamental in determining whether and how to treat a child: knowing how to differentiate a steaming related to growth, from a fever from wind or cold damage, is essential in deciding whether to abstain from treatment. Wrong decisions stemming from a lack of knowledge of these developmental stages can harm the vital essence of the child - negating the very purpose of medicine.

The chapters on birth and neonatal care are very exciting to me: they are very much in harmony with midwifery practices, even modern, and I was thrilled to find many useful new ideas as well as to recognize many age old techniques that defy time and geography. In my work with local midwives and pregnant, birthing and postpartum women, I often attend births and witness the early life of many babies, monitoring their umbilical cords, breastfeeding, digestion... the advice Sūn Sīmiǎo gives is so on point that it is undoubtable that he must have been present at many births himself. Some of the resuscitation techniques are very much on parr with some of the techniques we now use, preceding the administration of oxygen. The advice he gives regarding milk production, and digestive upset in newborns is extremely practical, combining immemorial midwifery knowledge about positioning the baby correctly to the nipple, feeding times and amounts etc, with a deep understanding of Jueyin-Yangming physiology. He emphasizes that some diseases of babies are a consequence of maternal deficiency, which is a vastly useful topic in the postpartum period when a practitioner has to care for the mother and the baby as a dyad.

Sūn Sīmiǎo also offers an in-depth discussion of conglomerations - their etiology, their consequences and their treatment. The proper elimination of such infantile aggregations is very important for the future health of the person in his eyes, and here again his perspective sheds a lot of light on this somewhat mysterious pathology, which has been the subject of many discussions through the ages.

Finally his chapter on seizures is most remarkable, differentiating many kinds of possible causes and presentations. As the mother of a child with epilepsy, as well as an avid student of the medical classics, I found this chapter most fascinating. In addition to some of the more well-know remedies of the *Shāng Hán Zá Bìng Lùn*, other recipes are given which are mind-blowing in their composition. Woven in the architecture of the formulae one can find the thinking of the Nei Jing, of Zhang Zhong Jing, Wang Shuhe and Tao Hong Jing... and furthering and confirming our thoughts Sūn

Sīmiǎo, humble and kind to his posterity despite the stature of his mind, makes sure to explain his understanding of the pathologies and formulae. What a gem in the treasury of medical literature!

This volume contains the essential foundations of pediatric medical knowledge upon which a practitioner must root him/herself and grow from. Sūn Sīmiǎo chose to organize his encyclopedia following the cycle of life, starting with women and continuing with children. In his title for the pediatric volume, "Nurturing the Root", is the quintessence of medicine. This title contains many layers of the same thought. In order to treat humanity we must start as young as before life is created (with the Mother); in order to have a healthy adult, and therefore healthy future generations, we must take great care of our young; and finally, both in the broadest and in the narrowest sense, our Root, at the cusp of Shaoyin, must be nurtured so that the cycle of life - whether circadian, physiological or cosmological, or all those levels at once - can perpetuate itself. Sūn Sīmiǎo achieves in his work the masterful feat of imparting his readers with an understanding of the creation and growth of Life, and giving them tools to cultivate it within themselves and others. His work fulfills the lofty daoist ideal of the study of life, while remaining highly practical and relevant to clinical practice. I am deeply grateful to Sabine Wilms for making this inspiring work widely available to the West!

Genevieve Le Goff, L.Ac.
Woodacre, CA.

How To Use This Book

The reader will find the literal English translation side-by-side with the Chinese text, augmented, where necessary, with explanatory notes. This gives the reader an opportunity to explore the Chinese text separately from the translation.

Since this publication offers the side-by-side comparison of the original Chinese text with the literal translation, the reader may notice that some of the titles in English do not have matching Chinese text. The translator has taken license by adding headings to many of the sections of the book. This is for ease of categorization and navigation. Also, this is not an unprecedented action on the part of the author. Many Chinese authors and scholars during the Sòng period also added in titles and headers where they saw fit.

Throughout the book the reader will find grey boxes. These boxes denote text and commentary that is not directly from the *Qiān Jīn Fāng*. The commentaries boxes written by Sabine Wilms and Brenda Hood are provided to give deeper insight around unusual terms or practices. There are also grey boxes after all major formulas or formula groups in the text that are identified as 千金方衍義 in the Chinese and as "Expanded Meaning" in the translation. These boxes constitute a literal translation of the entire *Qiān Jīn Fāng Yǎn Yì* 千金方衍義 ("Expanded Meaning of the Thousand Gold Prescriptions"), the only historical commentary on the *Bèi Jí Qiān Jīn Yào Fāng* that was composed by the famous scholar-physician Zhāng Lù 張璐. More information on this book and its author can be found in the translator's Introduction.

Acknowledgments

Thanks to all my students, past and present, from seasoned practitioners with a lifetime of experience to tentative first-year acupuncture students, for your interest in the history of your medicine, for your dedication and hard work in tackling classical Chinese, for peppering me with incisive questions that take me far outside my comfort zone, and most importantly for forcing me regularly to clarify to you and to myself why the ancient medical classics always have been and always should be an integral part of any Chinese medicine education. You remind me daily of how lucky I am to know what I know, teach what I teach, and translate what I translate, because it makes a difference in real people's lives.

Thanks to the infamous Rothenburg Three (Peter Firebrace, Lillian Pearl Bridges, and Debra Betts), for fun, friendship, music, and moral support when I really needed it; to Sunjae Lee for music, friendship, and art, most notably the gorgeous artwork that is gracing the cover of this book; and to Genevieve leGoff, for your open heart and inquisitive mind, selfless dedication to the medicine, and for being such a good mom; and to all the other lovely dedicated people in the academic and clinical worlds of Chinese medicine, for striving to make the world a better place. You are too many to name but you know who you are.

Thanks to my dear friends Brenda Hood and Kim Gray, without whose professional support, faith in this project, and selfless devotion Happy Goat Productions would not be producing anything. My eternal gratitude to both of you, for so much more than I could ever express.

Thanks to Wang Fengyi, Liu Lihong, Abbot Ming Chan, Heiner and Sheron Fruehauf, Laurie Regan, and Tamara Staudt, for forcing me to turn around and "venerate my roots" for the first time in my life last year at a retreat that changed my life and the direction of my work.

Thanks to my parents, for continuing to believe in me, through thick and thin.

Thanks to Lulu, Nilson, and Rose, the world's best dogs, for their unlimited bouncing joy and pure animal love.

Thanks to the great Oregon rainforest, and especially to that one special Devil's Club up on Larch Mountain, for holding me, reminding me of my roots, and putting everything in perspective.

Introduction

The Significance of Pediatrics

Based on extant medical writings from antiquity in both China and Europe, the proper care of newborns and young children was a topic that received far greater attention in early and medieval China than in Europe. To cite just one example, the *Yì Wén Zhì* 藝文志, a bibliographic treatise from the first century CE that details the holdings of the imperial library in the early Hàn period already lists a full nineteen volumes of formulas for women and children. By contrast, we find only short comments on individual diseases in Western medical literature by famous authors like Soranus of Ephesus (ca. 100 CE), Galen (ca. 200 CE), or Avicenna (ca. 990 CE), but no separate book-length treatises until Hieronymus published the first book on children's diseases in 1583. In the following centuries, writings on pediatrics became more common but there is no doubt that compared to other medical fields pediatrics is a very young specialty in the history of Western medicine. One could even argue that this attitude is still reflected in the lack of attention paid to pediatrics in modern TCM education in Western countries, especially when compared to Chinese medicine as practiced historically in China. It may therefore surprise even experienced practitioners of Chinese medicine who are unable to access the Chinese primary sources on their own, to learn of the emphasis placed on the care of women and children in the traditional Chinese medical literature.

The text that provides the source for the translation in the present book is a monumental encyclopedia of medicine called *Bèi Jí Qiān Jīn Yào Fāng*《備急千金要方》(Essential Formulas Worth a Thousand in Gold to Prepare for Emergencies) that was completed by Sūn Sīmiǎo in 652 CE, in the early Táng dynasty. While certainly a pathbreaking work in the history of Chinese pediatrics, its diagnostic and therapeutic advice did not appear out of nowhere but was firmly rooted in earlier texts, most of which have unfortunately not survived the vicissitudes of time. And the principles and treatments mentioned here were quickly expanded on and deepened in the following centuries, resulting in a whole body of literature on pediatrics when the field was established as a full-fledged medical specialization in the Imperial Bureau of Medicine during the Sòng dynasty. Sūn Sīmiǎo himself introduces the volume on pediatrics in the *Qiān Jīn Fāng* as follows:

> There is no *Dào* (lit. "path," but here in the sense of "skill" or "practice") among the common people that is greater than the *Dào* of nurturing the young. If [children] are not nurtured when they are young, they die before reaching adulthood. ... The present collection of treatments is arranged by placing the treatments for women and children first, and those for men and the elderly afterwards. The significance of this structure is that it venerates the root.
>
> Nevertheless, the force of qì is still feeble in small children, and medical gentlemen need to take great care to rescue and cure them and meritoriously offer their services to help them recover from serious conditions. The majority of present-day scholars fail to hold on to this intention. For this reason, when infants in swaddling clothes are concerned, surrounded by the foul stench of breast milk, how dare we look down on those doctors who carry out heroic acts?...
>
> ...At present, I have made abundant selections from amongst the various masters while also including effective treatments that I have personally experienced, to compose this chapter. Each and every household should master this "art of nurturing the young," so that it will be spared the calamity of untimely death....

In this context, the placement of the information on children right after the section on gynecology but ahead of the main part of the book that covers general medicine is highly significant. As Sūn Sīmiǎo himself stated unequivocally, this radical innovation and restructuring of medical information was not coincidental but on purpose. In his own words, he prioritized the health and welfare of women and children over those of other family members in order to "venerate the root.

Of all of Sūn Sīmiǎo's medical innovations, such as the introduction of Indian drugs and treatment methods, the first mention of the a-shi point (*ā shì xué* 阿是穴), the protocol of the so-called "thirteen ghost points" (*shí sān guǐ xué* 十三鬼穴), or his essay on medical ethics, his most important contribution to the history of Chinese medicine may well be this emphasis on gynecology and pediatrics as areas of special concern for any medically-oriented "specialist of nurturing life" (*yǎng shēng zhī jiā* 養生之家). The effects of this attitude can be seen to this day in the continuing significance of gynecology and pediatrics in Chinese medicine as practiced in contemporary China. Because of a lack of translations, however, this is an emphasis that has unfortunately not been recognized and utilized to its fullest potential in the application of Chinese medicine in non-Asian environments. It is my hope that the publication of this translation may serve as the beginning of a greater recognition of the potential role that traditional Chinese pediatrics can play in providing the best possible care for our children today. By making this ancient text accessible in English, I hope that practitioners worldwide will feel empowered and inspired to explore a field of Chinese medicine that is woefully neglected and underutilized at the moment by most practitioners of Chinese medicine in a non-Asian context.

Sūn Sīmiǎo, China's Greatest Doctor?

Whether native Chinese or foreign, medical historians, doctors of Chinese medicine, Daoist practitioners, and any other interested scholars or practitioners all agree that Sūn Sīmiǎo played a monumental role in the history of Chinese medicine. Depending on the individual's background, however, there is wide disagreement on the specific contributions that he is believed to have made. Modern TCM circles in both China and abroad revere him as one of China's greatest physicians who wholeheartedly dedicated himself to a life of serving the common people by selflessly treating local peasants and experimenting with the effect of medicinal substances on his own body. For practitioners of Daoism and *yǎng shēng* (養生, "nurturing life"), he is a source of inspiration as a recluse who lived in a secluded mountain cave on a diet of pine cones, mushrooms, and dew drops in the company of a tiger and a dragon until he transformed his body and attained immortality. Two accounts of his life are included in collections of biographies that are close enough to his lifetime as to be significant: The *Xù*

Xiān Zhuàn 《續仙傳》("Further Biographies of Immortals"), composed by Shěn Fén 沈汾 and cited in the 10th century Daoist encyclopedia *Yún Jí Qī Qiān* 《雲笈七籤》("Seven Bamboo Slips from a Cloud Satchel"), and, our earliest extant source, the *Huá Yán Jīng Chuán Jì* 《華嚴經傳記》("Records of the Transmission of the Avatamsaka Sutra"), composed by Fǎ Zàng 法藏 (643-712). While too terse to provide much information, we can take away the simple fact that Sūn Sīmiǎo was celebrated during the Táng dynasty as an immortal on the one hand, and a specialist in the Avatamsaka Sutra on the other. As the deified object of a cult to the "King of Medicinals" (*yào wáng* 藥王), lastly, he continues to be venerated especially on his purported birthday, the 28th day of the 4th lunar month, in a popular cult that Paul U. Unschuld has dated to the fourteenth or fifteenth century and that is still being actively promoted by local authorities for the sake of tourist money.

Legends about his life and work, purported treatments, heroic acts, and quotations from his writings abound in contemporary Chinese sources as much as in Western languages. Being the administrator of a Facebook page on Sūn Sīmiǎo and a lecturer on Sūn Sīmiǎo at large Chinese medicine conferences, I get asked constantly to confirm stories or quotations that I have never heard of even though I have spent much of my adult life studying Sūn Sīmiǎo and his writings. Although I may admire and want to support the spirit expressed in many of these accounts, my academic training as a critically-thinking historian forces me to abide by intellectual honesty and limit what I consider relevant information on Sūn Sīmiǎo to his own writings (if the determination of authorship is even possible in the context of medieval China) and to sources about him that were composed within several centuries of his lifetime.

Nathan Sivin has summarized the outcome of his research in what he considers historically solid knowledge on Sūn Sīmiǎo in this way: "In the case of Sun, our warrantable knowledge, based on the incontrovertible testimony of a well-placed witness, at least allows us to set him in his time: Sun was in the Emperor's retinue in 673, and stated at the time that he was born in 581; despite the great age which these dates imply, he was in excellent condition, body and mind. Nothing else survives the process of elimination.

My own approach is a bit less critical, motivated by the fact that I am not trying to reconstruct a detailed account of Sūn's life, for the simple reason that that is impossible. Rather, my interest in Sūn Sīmiǎo as a living person with a specific educational background and training, professional and social activities, and health-cultivation practices like diet, lifestyle, or exercises to move qì, is based on my desire to gain a sense of the cultural environment that produced the writings that we now celebrate as having been authored by the legendary figure we call Sūn Sīmiǎo. From that perspective, it is ultimately irrelevant whether he did in fact achieve immortality by consuming mercury or mounting 93 virgins without ejaculating, visited with dragon kings and demons, treated retained placenta by burning the husband's underwear, introduced Ayurvedic concepts or medicinal substances from India, or invented effective medicinal treatments for goiter or night blindness or malaria that satisfy modern scientific standards. What is relevant is that all these topics were considered essential aspects of medical practice in medieval China, important enough to have been included in the *Qiān Jīn Fāng* and thereby preserved for posterity.

In addition to his own writings, which I will discuss below, the two official biographies compiled by court historians several centuries after his death provide our only solid sources of information. In these biographies, Sūn Sīmiǎo emerges as a man of great intellectual talent, a youth prodigy with a standard literati education in the Classics, and a scholar with celebrated literary skills and deep insights into the Confucian, Buddhist, and Daoist literature. In addition, he was known as a master of highly technical esoteric matters, such as calendrical calculations, astrology, and physiognomy, able to read a variety of signs in the present in such a way as to discern developments in the future. Because of his uncompromising moral standards, he repeatedly declined invitations to serve as Erudite at court under immoral rulers such as Emperor Xuān of the Zhōu 周宣帝 (578-579) or Emperor Wén of the Suí 隋文帝 (580-589), instead choosing to live in obscurity until the reunification of China under the Táng dynasty and the emergence of a sage ruler. In 627 CE, he finally accepted an invitation to join the Táng emperor Tàizōng 太宗 as an advisor and then spent half a century at the imperial court. It is thus obvious that Sūn Sīmiǎo was a celebrated member of the highest elite in the early Táng dynasty, known for his erudition, moral standards, and sagely illumination, but also for his supernatural powers and cosmological insights. He was honored by the most powerful ruler in the world and surrounded himself with illustrious poets, calligraphers, politicians, philosophers, alchemists, and Buddhist and Daoist practitioners. After he was allowed to retire on the pretext of illness in the year 674, at almost 150 years of age if we read his biographies literally and place his birthdate in the late 520s, he disappears again into obscurity. It is generally agreed that his death occurred in 682 CE.

The most important fact about all accounts of Sūn Sīmiǎo's life that date to within a few centuries of his lifetime is the absence of any reference to medical practice. Nowhere do we find information on medical apprenticeships or a lineage, accounts of his medical activities, or records of successful treatments. The only mention of medicine at all is found in a conversation that Sūn Sīmiǎo is having with his disciple Lú Zhàolín 盧照鄰, one of the four great poets of the early Táng period. Suffering from an incurable disease, Lú asks his master not for a treatment or diagnosis but to explain to him the "principles used by the famous physicians to cure illness." Sūn Sīmiǎo is happy to oblige with a statement that is worth quoting in full here:

> I have heard that if one is skilled at talking about Heaven, one must substantiate it in the human realm; if one is skilled at talking about humans, one must also root it in Heaven. In Heaven, there are four seasons and five movements. Winter cold and summer heat alternate with each other. When this cyclical revolution is harmonious, it forms rain; when it is angry, wind; when it congeals, frost and snow; when it lengthens, rainbows. These are the constancies of Heaven and Earth.
>
> Humans have four limbs and five *zàng* organs. Alternating between being awake and sleeping, exhaling and inhaling and spitting out and sucking in, essence and qì come and go. In their flow, they constitute *yíng* provisioning and *wèi* defense; in their manifestation, they constitute the complexion; as they effuse to the surface, they constitute sound. These are the constancies of humanity. Yáng employs the outer form, yīn employs the essence, this is where Heaven and humanity are identical.

> As for losing them, steaming results in the generation of heat; stoppage results in the generation of cold; knotting together results in tumors and excrescences; caving in results in abscesses and ulcers; rushing results in panting and gasping; being used up results in parching and withering. The symptoms erupt on the face, and the changes stir the outer form.
>
> When one extends this analogy to apply to Heaven and Earth, it is likewise. Thus the waxing and waning of the five planets, the irregular motions of the constellations, the eclipses of the sun and moon, the flight of shooting stars, these are Heaven and Earth's symptoms of danger. Unseasonable winter cold and summer heat are the steaming up or standstill of Heaven and Earth. Uprighted boulders and thrust-up earth are the tumors and excrescences of Heaven and Earth; landslides or collapsing ground are the abscesses and ulcers of Heaven and Earth; windstorms and torrential rains are the panting and gasping of Heaven and Earth. Dried up rivers and ditches are the parching and withering of Heaven and Earth.
>
> An excellent physician guides [disease out of the body] by means of medicinals and [lancing] stones and rescues by means of needles and prescriptions. A sage harmonizes [Heaven and Earth] with consummate virtue and supports them by means of human affairs. Thus, the human body has illnesses that can be cured, and Heaven and Earth have calamities that can be dispersed.

I quote this statement here in a literal translation because it is in fact a beautiful summary of the deep connection between medicine and politics, between the human and the cosmic realms, expressed most vividly in what is known in English as "correlative thinking" through the vehicles of yīn-yáng and the five dynamic movements (*yīn yáng wǔ xíng* 陰陽五行). This macrocosmic dimension is, I believe, of fundamental importance if we are to fully appreciate the significance and connotations of Sūn Sīmiǎo's medical writings, or of any medical discourse in classical China in general. While perhaps more obvious in philosophical treatises like the *Huáng Dì Nèi Jīng* 《黃帝內經》(Yellow Emperor's Inner Classic) than in formulary literature, for example, the equivalence and mutual influence of all sorts of microcosms, from the human body to the family, politics, and natural cycles, on each other and on the macrocosm at large is such an ingrained aspect of classical Chinese thinking that it often went unspoken but was never absent. It is the reason why we find, for example, a detailed description of the development of the fetus among the famous Mǎwángduī manuscripts that date from before 168 BCE. It is obviously also an excellent reason why Sūn Sīmiǎo in his role as advisor to the emperor should have been so interested in the art of "nurturing the small," a skill that any careful and conscientious ruler would be bound to appreciate.

"Nurturing Life" (*yǎng shēng* 養生) by "Nurturing the Small" (yǎng xiǎo 養小): The Connection Between Macrobiotic Hygiene and Pediatrics in the *Qiān Jīn Fāng*

Nevertheless, the extent of Sūn Sīmiǎo's emphasis on the care of women and children over any other aspect of medicine suggests that his interest was peeked by more than just the political value and cosmological significance of promoting the feminine, yīn, or the giver of life in the case of women, and the small, vulnerable, stage of inception, birth, at its most yáng stage, in the case of newborn children. For a more complete answer, let us look at Sūn Sīmiǎo's actual writings. There is no doubt that the *Qiān Jīn Fāng* is a central text in the history of Chinese medicine. A gigantic encyclopedia, its thirty volumes contain over five thousand entries in the form of *fāng* 方 ("formulas," "recipes," or "prescriptions" in the largest sense of that word, but literally meaning "directions") and occasional short essays. These *fāng* cover a large range of therapeutic approaches, representative of all that was considered medicine (*yī* 醫) in medieval China: internal medications (medicinal decoctions, powders, pills, pastes, jellies, or liquors), external treatments (ointments, plasters, hot compresses and suppositories, fumigations, baths, beauty treatments, physical manipulations, and acupuncture and moxibustion), religious methods (talismans, exorcistic rituals, spells, and incantations) and what we might call lifestyle advice (exercise, diet, sexual intercourse, avoidance of stress and overwork, etc.).

Even a cursory look at the outline of the *Qiān Jīn Fāng* reveals that Sūn Sīmiǎo organized his information in a way that differs dramatically from contemporaneous medical texts: The famous formula collection *Jīn Guì Yào Lüè* 《金匱要略》 ("Essential Prescriptions of the Golden Cabinet," Eastern Hàn period) covers women's conditions at the very end of the general section, followed only by a brief section on "miscellaneous formulas" and dietetics that most scholars believe to have been added to the original text in the Sòng period, and has nothing at all to say about pediatrics. Another text, composed only decades before the *Qiān Jīn Fāng* but clearly influential for Sūn Sīmiǎo's thinking, the *Zhū Bìng Yuán Hòu Lùn* 《諸病源候論》("On the Origins and Signs of the Various Diseases," 610) covers pediatrics in the very end, following right after the information on gynecology in the last six of fifty volumes. What is significant in this context, however, is not that pediatrics is placed at the very end of the text but that over a tenth of the total text is devoted to this topic. Its author, Cháo Yuánfāng, served as officially-appointed imperial physician and erudite in the Suí dynasty court. Following a similar structure and weight, the *Wài Tái Mì Yào* 《外臺祕要》("Classified Secrets From the Palace Library," 752), another formula collection that was published slightly later than the *Qiān Jīn Fāng*, covers the prevention and treatment of pediatric diseases in volumes 35 and 36 out of 40, right after volumes 33-34 on gynecology, recording about 400 formulas in 86 chapters. We can therefore presume that pediatrics was a topic near and dear to the heart of not just Sūn Sīmiǎo as an individual but of medically-inclined writers and practitioners during the early Táng period in general.

The important role pediatrics played in medieval Chinese medicine is further confirmed a few centuries later by its official recognition in terms of publications and institutional structures in the imperial medical bureau of the Sòng dynasty. This initial stage of pediatrics culminated in 1119 with the publication of the *Xiǎo Ér Yào Zhèng Zhí Jué* 《小兒藥証直訣》(Straight Tricks on Medicinals and Signs in Pediatrics) in three volumes, composed by the famous pediatrician Qián Yǐ 錢乙 after more than forty years of gathering clinical experience and academic research. The first volume, titled "Pulses, Signs, and Treatment Methods," discusses information on physiology, pathology, five *zàng* organ-based disease differentiation, and 80 disease patterns. Volume two, titled "Case Histories," presents Qián Yǐ's personal clinical experience in 23 case histories; volume three, on "Various Formulas," presents essential pediatric formulas and introduces 122 of Qián Yǐ's own most effective formulas. As the preface to his book states (my paraphrase), medicine is already a difficult art, but pediatrics is particularly difficult for the following reasons: First, not much information is recorded in the classics. Second, children's pulses are difficult to read and small children (here defined as below the age of seven) easily wail from fright, forcing the physician to rely on outside signs. Third, their bones, qì, body shape, and voice are not yet fully developed and they often behave abnormally, whether crying in sadness or laughing in joy. 4) Small children cannot speak yet or their words are unreliable, so it is impossible to gain information by questioning them. 5) Children's internal organs are weak and thus susceptible to vacuity or repletion or heat or cold. In addition, ordinary physicians carelessly prescribe substances like *xījiǎo* (rhinoceros horn), *zhēnzhū* (pearl), *lónggǔ*, and *shèxiāng*, complicating the condition. For this reason, ordinary physician's kill four out of ten patients by mistreatment.

This brief review demonstrates that the diagnostic and therapeutic sophistication of Chinese pediatricians like Qián Yǐ, reflected in transmitted medical literature from the seventh century on, was light-years ahead of any parallel developments in European medicine. The question now becomes: What stimulated this rise in interest in the care of women and children and subsequent development of gynecology and pediatrics as respected and highly valued medical specializations from the Sòng period on? For potential answers, it behooves us to return to Sūn Sīmiǎo and the *Qiān Jīn Fāng*. As already mentioned above, the arrangement of medical information in this seminal text is a significant change from formula collections with similar content, and it is therefore helpful to take a closer look at the structure of the book. Its thirty scrolls cover the following content in a total of thirty volumes:

Volume 1: Preface
Sūn Sīmiǎo's famous essays on medical ethics and medical education, plus general information on treatment principles, diagnostics, guidelines for writing prescriptions, individual medicinals, combining medicinals, contraindications, and medicinal storage

Volume 2: Gynecology I
Fertility, pregnancy, obstetrics, and lactation

Volumes 3-4: Gynecology II
Postpartum depletion, wind strike, supplementation, vaginal discharge, menstrual disorders, and other gynecological conditions

Volume 5: Pediatrics

Volume 6: Diseases of the seven orifices
I.e., mouth, nose, eyes, lips, teeth, throat, ears, and facial treatments

Volume 7: Wind poison foot qì
I.e., wind poison invading the body through the feet

Volume 8: Various wind disorders

Volumes 9-10 : Cold damage

Volumes 11-20: Diseases of the internal organs
Liver, gallbladder, heart, small intestine, spleen, stomach, lung, large intestine, kidney, and bladder respectively

Volume 21: Fluid metabolism
Dispersion thirst, strangury, hematuria, and water swelling

Volume 22: Skin conditions
Ulcers, sores, swelling, eczema, etc.

Volume 23: Hemorrhoids and fistulas

Volume 24: Resolving poisons and miscellaneous other treatments

Volume 25: Emergencies

Volume 26: Dietetics

Volume 27: "Nurturing the Inner Nature,"
i.e. reclusive life, alchemy, massage, qì cultivation, sexual cultivation, various prohibitions

Volume 28: Pulse diagnosis

Volumes 29-30: Acupuncture and moxibustion

As Sūn Sīmiǎo himself points out in the introduction to the volume on pediatrics that I have already quoted above, "The present collection of treatments is arranged by placing the treatments for women and children first, and those for men and the elderly afterwards. The significance of this structure is that it venerates the root." This short and innocuous statement is Sūn's only stated explanation and explicit reference to the unconventional structure of his book, but it truly does provide a clear and reasonable answer. We can flesh out Sūn's intention with the little we know about his life from the historical accounts summarized above, in combination with other statements of his in the *Qiān Jīn Fāng*, especially in his treatise on medical ethics (in volume 1) and a number of passages in volume 27 on "Nurturing the Inner Nature" (*yǎng xìng* 養性).

To summarize the information about Sūn Sīmiǎo and his values found in historical sources within a few centuries of his lifetime, two factors stand out that are relevant to the topic at hand: First, Sūn Sīmiǎo was a man of outstanding virtue, deeply rooted in and affected by classical Chinese values expressed in the Confucian, Daoist, and Buddhist literature that he not only studied but also actively cultivated throughout his life. While not preserved independently, his accomplishments in areas like calligraphy, poetry, philosophy, and politics were widely respected and recognized by the highest levels of the early Táng elite. Second, the long periods of reclusion in his life in combination with his longevity (or immortality, depending on the account) and mastery of other seemingly superhuman skills caused his contemporaries to associate him with the realm of *shén xiān* 神仙 ("immortals"). As such, he was a devoted student of the "technical skills of nurturing life"(*yǎng shēng zhī shù* 養生之術, *Qiān Jīn Fāng* I.8), which he apparently applied to his own body with great success. From a modern Western perspective, the connection between medicine and personal experimentation with natural substances, qì-cultivation (whether through breath, meditation, diet, or exercises), sexual intercourse, or divination by means of face reading, yarrow stalks, or astrology may not be immediately obvious. But in the medieval Chinese context, it makes perfect sense.

In my eyes, Sūn Sīmiǎo's greatest contribution lies in this powerful combination of medicine with moral cultivation and physical cultivation. To give just a few examples, he states in volume 27 on "Nurturing the Inner Nature" (*yǎng xìng* 養性): "If a person's virtue in actions is not abundant, even if they constantly take elixirs of jade and pills of gold, they will be unable to extend their longevity." And further below in the same chapter, "A person who is skilled at preserving life will not encounter ferocious tigers. This is heaven's reward for having morality (*dào dé* 道德)." It is only natural that Sūn's dedication to this *dào dé*, what we might call "ethics" or "morality" for lack of a better English translation, to fulfilling one's individual human responsibility to carry out the *Dào* of Heaven, also affected how he viewed medical practice. His essay on medical ethics in volume 1 of the *Qiān Jīn Fāng* reflects a melding of Buddhist, Daoist, and Confucian values that is a unique characteristic of medieval Chinese culture and has been appreciated worldwide as a key contribution to the history of medical ethics. Allow me to quote a short excerpt.

> In all cases, when you treat disease as a "great physician," you must quiet your spirit and fix your intention, you must be free of wants and desires, and you must first develop a heart full of great compassion and empathy. You must pledge your desire to rescue all sentient beings indiscriminately from their suffering. If someone facing disease or disaster comes to you seeking relief, you may not inquire whether the person is nobility or low class or poor or wealthy, [or consider their] old age or youth, beauty or ugliness, or whether you detest or like them or whether they are your friend, whether they are Chinese or barbarian, a fool or a sage. You must treat all of them exactly the same as if they were your closest relatives. Neither must you look to the front while turning around to cover your back, worry about your personal fortune or misfortune, and guard and cherish your own life. When seeing the suffering and grief of others, you must act as if it were your own and open your heart deeply to their misery. You must not avoid dangerous mountains with rugged cliffs, any time of day or night, the cold of winter or heat of summer, hunger or thirst, fatigue and exhaustion. You must focus your heart on attending to their rescue and must not have a heart of hard labor or outward appearances. Acting like this, you can serve as eminent physician for the masses; acting against this, you are a horrid thief to all sentient beings…
>
> Lord Lao said: "When humans carry out acts of visible virtue, humans will reciprocate on their own; when humans carry out acts of hidden virtue, the spirits will reciprocate. When humans carry out acts of visible vice, humans will reciprocate on their own; when humans carry out acts of hidden vice, the spirits will harm them. For this reason, as physician you may not depend on your own greatness [alone] and focus your heart on official ranks and material possessions, but you must create a heart intent on relieving suffering.

> Then, in the midst of experiencing the obscurity of your fate, you will yourself feel blessed in multiple ways.

How did this way of thinking, these views on medicine, ethics, and self-cultivation, affect Sūn Sīmiǎo's attitude towards pediatrics? The most logical explanation in my mind, though never spelled out by Sūn Sīmiǎo or his contemporaries, hinges on the meaning of the term *yǎng shēng*, referenced consistently throughout the *Qiān Jīn Fāng*. Usually translated literally and quite adequately as "nurturing life," the etymology of the two separate characters that make up the term might shed some light on what the early Chinese had in mind when they used the term. The character *shēng* 生 is fairly straight-forward: It is an image of a plant emerging from the ground, a sprout in the early stage of growth. Hence it means "life," "birth," "generation" in addition to its narrowest meaning of "sprouting." As such, it is used twice, for example, in a classic line from *Sù Wèn*《素問》5, first to refer to the first of the four stages of development in nature throughout the four seasons and second to the verb "produce" or "engender": 天有四時五行，以生長收藏，以生寒暑燥濕風。"Heaven has four seasons and five movements, whereby it causes birth, growth, gathering, and storing, and whereby it engenders cold, summer-heat, dryness, dampness, and wind." We can see how in both contexts the metaphor of "sprouting" fits quite well. The first character in the compound *yǎng shēng* is perhaps even more evocative: *yǎng* 養 is a combination of 羊, the image of a sheep, the quintessential sacrificial animal, hence here conveying the notion of sacrifice to the spirits or one's ancestors, and 食, a character denoting "food" or "feeding." As a combination of these two components, the character *yǎng* 養 hence referred originally to the concept of offering food in sacrifice to one's ancestral spirits. From there, it came to mean "nourishing," "nurturing," "supporting," "cultivating," or even "rearing" in the context of animal husbandry. On the most general level, perhaps "providing for" or "offering sustenance" are good renditions.

So how might we use the concept of *yǎng shēng* to explain Sūn Sīmiǎo's unusual emphasis on the care of women and children and radical break with literary tradition? As he himself stated, after all, "The diseases of small children are no different from those of adults. The only difference lies in the quantity of medicinals that are used. The eight or nine chapters on fright seizures, intrusive upset, separated skull, failure to walk, etc. are here combined into the present volume. Other treatments for conditions like diarrhea etc. are scattered throughout the various other volumes [of the *Qiān Jīn Fāng*] and can be found there." Viewed at from this angle, it surely would make more sense to follow tradition and explain the care of the human body in general, regardless of gender or age differences, first, before delving into specialized conditions. Nevertheless, as soon as we translate the term *yǎng shēng* literally as "providing for sprouting," and recall the centrality of this notion in Sūn Sīmiǎo's life and work, the answer is clear. I therefore propose that Sūn Sīmiǎo consciously broke with literary tradition and placed the formulas for women and children in the front of the general section to emphasize the importance of "venerating the root," of truly and literally supporting the process of life in its entirety by beginning with the generation and sprouting. The extent of Sūn Sīmiǎo's clinical experience may always remain a mystery, at least to critical historians like myself, but the more I study Master Sūn's writings, the more that question becomes a mute point. More important to me is Sūn Sīmiǎo's very real and explicit sensitivity to the fragility of life at its inception, yet another expression of his sagely insights into the transformations of qì in the natural cycles of life, in the macrocosm of heaven and earth as much as in the microcosm of the human body."

Sūn Sīmiǎo's Writings on Pediatrics: Summary of Content

The introduction to volume 5 of the *Qiān Jīn Fāng* on pediatrics begins with the following statement: "Among the methods for engendering humans (*shēng rén zhī dào* 生人之道), none fail to constitute the big by means of nurturing the small. Without attention to the small, death ensues before the big is completed. For this reason, the *Yì Jīng*《易經》("Classic of Changes") says: '[Enable] that which is small to come together so as to complete that which is big....'" Motivated by this recognition of the importance of "nurturing the small," Sūn Sīmiǎo then proceeded to provide all the relevant information he was able to find on the proper care of neonates, infants and young children. The information in these pages strikes a useful balance between his repeatedly stated preference for "treating disease before it arises" (*zhì wèi bìng* 治未病)

and his desire to address the real practical needs of his readers to "prepare for critical situations" (*bèi jí* 備急), as the title of the *Qiān Jīn Fāng* proclaims, or in other words, between preventative care and the treatment of existing disease. The present book is a translation of the first half of volume 5, covering the first four of a total of nine chapters. In 12 essays, 47 formulas, 12 other methods, 24 moxibustion instructions, 2 incantations, and 1 technique for diagnosing seizures, Sūn Sīmiǎo addresses the topics of neonatal development, transformations and steamings, and the selection of a wet nurse (chapter 1), neonatal care, i.e., swaddling, cutting the cord, feeding, bathing, assessing neonatal health, prognosis, etc. (chapter 2), and the treatment of fright seizures (chapter 3) and "intrusive upset" (chapter 4). This is followed by another five chapters on: Cold Damage; Cough; Aggregations, Binds, Distention, and Fullness; Welling Abscesses, Flat Abscesses, and Scrofula; and "Miscellaneous Diseases" (chapters 5-9, respectively), containing an additional 242 formulas, 1 essay, and 15 moxibustion methods.

Compared to other volumes in the *Qiān Jīn Fāng*, the pediatrics section stands out for the following reason: With the exception of volume 1 (the introduction to the whole *Qiān Jīn Fāng*) and the volumes at the very end of the *Qiān Jīn Fāng* on dietetics, yǎng xìng, pulse diagnosis, and acupuncture and moxibustion, volume 5 contains a substantial number of essays, which tend to cover advice on basic infant care, preventative measures, and diagnostic guidelines. Without reading too much into this formal observation, we can speculate that this might reflect a greater focus on preventative care and early diagnosis in pediatrics than in other fields of medicine. This was perhaps related to the fact that the health of small children is so fragile and the treatment of pediatric conditions so complicated that medicinal formulas or moxibustion might have often been a case of too little too late, or on the contrary of further worsening a "dis-eased" state by inappropriate or overly aggressive treatment. To repeat here the frequent warnings found in the *Qiān Jīn Fāng* and all other pediatric literature in traditional China, children's bodies are weak and they are not fully developed in either physiology or anatomy, in addition to which they are more susceptible to invasion of external pathogens and respond more strongly. Sūn Sīmiǎo himself stresses the vulnerability of small children over and over, such as in the chapter on fright seizures:

> When babies first emerge from [the mother's] abdomen, the blood vessels are not drawn in and the five *zàng* organs are not yet matured. [At this point, even] slightly inappropriate care and nurturance immediately causes disease. Frequently, [such babies] will not reach adulthood...
>
> Right after babies are born, their birth qì is still exuberant. Nevertheless, if they do have some minor malignity, you must move it down [and out]. [In the course of this treatment,] you must not injure them in any way, and their recovery from the disease will thereby obtain the deepest benefit. If you fail to move [the illness] downward in time, it will mature into a major illness, and once that illness has matured, it will be difficult to treat indeed!

Rather than repeating here more information from the translation in the following pages and risking an interpretation of passages out of context, I ask the reader to study my translation as a whole.

Organization, Content, and Intention of this Translation

Much thought has gone into the layout, structure, components, and intentions of this translation project. It is informed by my three professional roles as an academic translator and producer of books on Chinese medicine; teacher of clinical content, medical literature, and classical Chinese; and practitioner of classical Chinese medicine in the largest sense of the term. I have spent years exploring with clinicians, academics, students, and fellow teachers what the best format may be for making classical medical writing accessible to a contemporary Western audience. The present book is the result of these conversations and the feedback I have received.

A critical reader might well question the basic premise of this whole project, namely the value of translating a text that predated what most historians of Chinese medicine consider the origin of Chinese pediatrics by several centuries. Why choose this volume from the *Qiān Jīn Fāng*, authored by a scholar, philosopher, and practitioner of *yǎng shēng* with no historically validated clinical experience himself, over a text like the *Xiǎo Ér Yào Zhèng Zhí Jué* 《小兒藥証直訣》(Straight Tricks on Medicinals and Signs in

Pediatrics) in three volumes, composed by the famous pediatrician Qián Yǐ 錢乙 in 1119 as the culmination of forty years of clinical practice? Or the *Yòu Yòu Xīn Shū* 《幼幼新書》 ("New Writings on Early Childhood"), a monumental text in 40 volumes that was compiled by an editorial team under Liú Fǎng 劉昉 in 1150 to comprehensively present all information on pediatrics available at the time? Or far easier still, why not simply translate the most modern, most advanced top-of-the-line textbook on TCM pediatrics from China, which would offer the highest standards of TCM pediatric knowledge as practiced today in modern China (besides being far easier to translate)? As sorely needed as such translations are and as clinically useful as they doubtlessly are as well, I have chosen to focus on Sūn Sīmiǎo's work for the following reasons:

Because I am a medical historian who specializes in pre-Sòng medical literature, I have my head in the classics all day long and am more familiar with classical Chinese of the early Táng and with medical literature in particular than most other translators, medical or otherwise. I treat Sūn Sīmiǎo's writings with the utmost reverence and am confronted almost daily with misinterpretations, mistranslations, or directly fabricated misinformation about who he was and what he might have said or done. While everybody agrees on the significance of Sūn Sīmiǎo's writings, there is so little solid information available in non-Asian languages, and the *Qiān Jīn Fāng* is such a difficult text to read for people without the proper training in classical Chinese of the early Táng period that we could fill a whole book with stories and myths about Sūn Sīmiǎo. Attractive and entertaining and perhaps even inspiring as they might be, they generally fail to be realistically related to Sūn Sīmiǎo's actual life and work. In my opinion, Sūn's actual vision of medicine and of each of our individual responsibility for and involvement with healing, of ourselves, of our families and relations, and of the universe at large, is far deeper than anything that anybody else could have invented about him.

Related to this point, there is no doubt that medical authors from the Sòng period on enjoyed much better access to resources than what would have been available to Sūn Sīmiǎo in the early Táng. Deeply committed to improving medicine as a means to provide for the welfare of the population, the Sòng court actively supported medical research, education, and training. It therefore provided large teams of scholars with what must have been the most comprehensive collections of medical literature in the world and with all the material support to carry out years of textual research in large editorial teams. And yet, to this day the vast majority of medical authors in contemporary China continue to liberally quote treatment principles and formulas from the *Qiān Jīn Fāng* to support their approach and root their insights in concepts and expressions from the classical literature. Classical Chinese pediatrics is a field that is in dire need of research and solid publications in Western languages, for the sake not only of Chinese Medicine practitioners and their little patients, but also of medical historians and other researchers. As the following pages will hopefully demonstrate, the fact that pediatrics did not exist yet as a separate medical field during Sūn's lifetime is no valid reason to ignore the insights expressed in the *Qiān Jīn Fāng* regarding preventative care, diagnosis, and treatment.

This book is intended primarily to address the need of contemporary practitioners of Chinese medicine for deeper and historically accurate information on the care of children in classical Chinese medicine. Continuing what I regard as a very healthy and important trend in recent Chinese medicine publications in the English language, I have chosen to present the literal English translation side-by-side with the Chinese text, augmented, where necessary, with explanatory notes. After years of attempting to introduce the treasure of classical Chinese medical literature to students and practitioners through my translations and live teaching, I become more convinced every day that no translation in a modern language can ever adequately express the range and depth of meaning found in the original source text in classical Chinese. Even very limited exposure to classical Chinese can deepen one's understanding of a difficult line with multiple dimensions of meaning that could never be expressed in English without a large explanatory comment. It is my sincere hope that more and more serious Chinese medicine students, regardless of their years of clinical experience, will rise to the challenge of studying the language in order to gain a better understanding of the classical roots of their medicine. May this book serve as the first step in bridging the gulf between our modern practice and the wisdom in the ancient texts.

My translation was done from a source text that I have created by collating a number of modern critical Chinese editions. The Chinese scholars who created these texts in turn based their research on the following editions of the *Qiān Jīn Fāng*:

1. A first woodblock print edition was published by the imperial Office for the Correction of Medical Literature (*jiào zhèng yī shū jú* 校正醫書局) under the direction of Lín Yì 林億 in the 1060s as part of the Sòng government's efforts to promote medical care by republishing corrected versions of the classics. A copy of this edition was discovered in Japan in the early nineteenth century and has been republished numerous times since then in China, Japan, and elsewhere.

2. Another version of the *Qiān Jīn Fāng* is found as part of the Daoist Canon (*Dào Zàng* 道藏), titled *Sūn Zhēn Rén Bèi Jí Qiān Jīn Yào Fāng*《孫真人備急千金要方》("Essential Prescriptions Worth a Thousand in Gold to Prepare for Emergencies by the Perfected Sūn). It appears to predate the Sòng revisions but suffers from numerous textual corruptions that reflect the Daoist slant of its editors. This is the version that was incorporated into the *Sì Kù Quán Shū*《四庫全書》encyclopedia.

3. Quotations appear in other received literature, most notably in the *Wài Tái Mì Yào*《外臺祕要》("Classified Secrets From the Palace Library," from 752) and the *Yī Xīn Fāng*《醫心方》("Prescriptions From the Heart of Medicine," from 984).

In addition, I have consulted a modern Chinese published version of a Sòng period manuscript that was discovered in 1799 and shows numerous discrepancies with any received versions based on the revisions by the Sòng editorial team under Lín Yì. Scholars therefore tend to date this text slightly earlier than the Sòng woodblock edition. The modern edition I have used is titled *Sūn Zhēn Rén Qiān Jīn Fāng*《孫真人千金方》("Thousand Gold Prescriptions by the Perfected Sūn") and was published in 1995 by Rén Mín Wèi Shēng 人民衛生 publishing house.

To make the text more accessible to clinically-oriented readers, we have chosen to supplement my translation and explanatory notes with two commentaries: We were fortunate to receive some clinical pearls from Dr. Brenda Hood, composed specifically for the purpose of this project in response to the text. Dr. Hood is one of the finest practitioners of Chinese medicine alive who combines an outstanding mastery of classical and modern medical Chinese with the most advanced TCM training from China and years of clinical experience. Furthermore, her doctoral research in Daoist and Buddhist self-cultivation literature and practices has given her a sensitivity to precisely the kinds of texts and practices that Sūn Sīmiǎo lived with and drew inspiration from.

Second, the present book includes a full translation of the pediatric section from the only historical commentary on the *Qiān Jīn Fāng*, the *Qiān Jīn Fāng Yǎn Yì* 《千金方衍義》("Expanded Meaning of the Thousand Gold Prescriptions"). Composed by the famous scholar-physician Zhāng Lù 張璐 who lived from 1617 to ca. 1700 during the transition from the Míng to the Qīng dynasties, it is a 30-volume text that the author completed in 1698 towards the end of a long and productive life of medical practice and research. Its earliest extant version dates from 1801 and constitutes the textual source for such modern editions as the one used for this book project, a 1995 edition by *Zhōng Guó Zhōng Yī Yào* 中國中醫藥. Zhāng Lù's commentary provides explanations for all major medicinal formulas in the *Qiān Jīn Fāng*, based on his many decades of clinical experience and textual studies of the medical literature. Known as one of the "Three Great Doctors of the Early Qīng" and a member of the School of Warming and Supplementing (*wēn bǔ pài* 温補派), his writings reflect a persistent interest in Cold Damage (*shāng hán* 傷寒) theory and influenced the development of Warm Disease (*wén bìng* 温病) theory in the Qīng period. In Zhāng Lù's eyes, no other figure in the history of Chinese medicine matched Zhāng Zhòngjǐng besides Sūn Sīmiǎo. Aware that nobody before him had dared to comment on and explain the *Qiān Jīn Fāng* because of its abstruse nature, he explained his motivation for taking on this formidable task in his preface: "If nobody were to elucidate this book and future generations would eventually fail to know of its existence, this would be deeply regrettable." The present publication is yet another attempt to prevent future generations from losing sight of it.

In terms of my choice of terminology and translation style, this project constitutes a literal translation and uses Nigel Wiseman's terminology, as published in his *Practical Dictionary of Chinese Medicine* (Nigel Wiseman and Feng Ye, Paradigm Publications, 1998), with exceptions noted and explained in the Translator's Notes throughout the text. For information on weights and measurements, please consult the chart on page 293 in this book.

The present book is a translation of the first half of Volume 5 on Pediatrics, to be followed shortly by the second half (on Cold Damage, Cough, Abdominal Masses and Digestive Issues, Abscesses, and Miscellaneous Diseases in Early Childhood). It is the first in a series of publications by Happy Goat Productions that aims at introducing Sūn Sīmiǎo's work to a Western audience. Other forthcoming publications will cover the following subjects:

- Background information on the *Qiān Jīn Fāng* and on Sūn Sīmiǎo;
- A volume dedicated to the materia medica of the *Qiān Jīn Fāng* with information on all medicinal substances used by Sūn Sīmiǎo, which will include a translation of all *Shén Nóng Běn Cǎo Jīng* entries;
- Translations of other volumes in the *Qiān Jīn Fāng*, most notably those on gynecology, nurturing life, dietetics, and the preface.

父母的心就是兒女的身，兒女的身就是父母的心。

"The heart of the parent is the body of the child;
the body of the child is the heart of the parent."
Liu Yousheng, Yanjianglu p. 160

Venerate The Root!

A mini-version of Sun Simiao's Qian Jin Fang chapter 5
by Peter Firebrace

Venerate the root! says Sun Simiao
Women and children first, that's my kind of *dao*!
Follow the art of *yang xiao*, nurturing the small
Get the beginnings right, so they stand up straight and tall!
Yes, ten months have passed since the moment of conception
But life's still fragile at its inception
Take good care now! Pay more attention, not less!
Nurture the young to avoid untimely death!
The Yijing, the Shijing, they all say the same thing!
There's nothing more important than getting off to a good start
Treatment of children is an essential part of a doctor's art!
In the small child the force of qi is still feeble
But you can help it along with herbs, moxibustion and needles!

So I've been listening, I've been gathering, collecting all the wisdom I can!
And I've set it all down to share with you
Theory, diagnostics, advice, effective treatments too
To help that little baby become a healthy woman or healthy man!
Normal development unfolds through *bian zheng*,
transformation and steaming
That gets the qi and blood growing, flowing, thriving and streaming!
This steaming heat and transforming rising qi
Come in definite phases, so let them be!
Keep the baby calm and rested, not a lot of people crowding around
Stay with them and observe them, that's how the answers can be found!
I'll tell you what's normal, I'll tell you what's not
Heat's OK, but not if the ears and buttocks are hot!
Then I'll give you the treatments you need to use
To bring them back to health, so the child you don't lose!
By the newborn's 288th day
Nine transformations and four steamings will have passed their way
For unresolved heat and phlegm, remember the Purple Pill, Zi Wan!
And in seasonal warmth complications, use the Black Powder, Hei San!
But don't be reckless with acupuncture, moxibustion or medicinals
Understand what's a normal process and what's pathological!

Directly after birth, keep the baby's mouth and tongue clean
Carefully wipe away any muck and blood to be seen
Check the newborn's not silent, take care cutting the cord
Cold, wind and dirt getting in, they can ill afford!
Take care of their delicate skin, when you're wrapping and swaddling
But expose them to mild, warm weather too!
They won't withstand wind and cold with too much molly-coddling

Their future health is down to you!
Wrap the umbilicus properly and ensure that it's healing
Follow my advice if it's infected, swollen or oozing!
From bathing to breast feeding, under or overeating
The child needs to be nurtured and protected
In thrush, connected tongue, sudden neonatal death and abscesses
There are treatments if the child's been affected
For diagnosis and prognosis, even its character and how long the baby will live
There are numerous tell-tale signs that the body gives!

Study *jing* seizures from fright, wind and food
Know when and when not to treat, how to get qi and blood renewed!
Avoid causing problems with inappropriate medicines or doses
Each have their sign and symptom picture, each have their own process!
Differentiate the five organ types, the six animal types, the time of day
Use moxibustion or a Gentian Decoction, a Rhubarb Decoction, maybe a Cinnamon Twig Decoction to get health back on its way!

Young children are sensitive, even vulnerable on occasion
In danger from the qi of strangers, from alien qi invasion
This is the pattern of intrusive upset *ke wu*
And it's important to know just what to do!
They get overwhelmed by 'visiting hostility'
And in this danger from strangers lose their self-protective ability!
Guard against exposure, keep them safe from intrusion!
Learn the moxibustion points, the spells, the herbal infusions!

To treat night crying and demonic possession, use shamanic solutions!

Children are the future, the roots that will be fruits
Take good care of them, like delicate flowers and shoots!
Understand their nature and treat them right
And the future that's unfolding will be strong and clear and bright!

Shào Xiǎo Yīng Rú Fāng

卷五：少小嬰孺方

VOLUME 5: TREATMENTS FOR SMALL CHILDREN AND INFANTS

PART 1

Preface
Emergence of the Newborn from the Abdomen
Fright Seizures
Intrusive Upset

Chapter One: Preface
序例第一

(5 paragraphs, 2 formulas, essay on "Selecting a Wet Nurse" attached)

論曰:

（一）夫生民之道，莫不以養小為大。

（二）若無於小，卒不成大。故《易》稱積小以成大；《詩》有厥初生民；《傳》云聲子生隱公。

（三）此之一義，即是從微至著，自少及長，人情共見，不待經史。

（四）故今斯方，先婦人、小兒，而後丈夫、耆老者，則是崇本之義也。

（五）然小兒氣勢微弱，醫士欲留心救療，立功瘥難。

（六）今之學者，多不存意，良由嬰兒在於襁褓之內，乳氣腥臊，醫者操行英雄，詎肯瞻視。

（七）靜而言之，可為太息者矣。

I.1 Essay

Line I.1.1

(1) Among the *Dàos*[1] of engendering humans, none fail to nurture the small to constitute the big. Without [care] for the small, death ensues before the big is completed.

(2) For this reason, the *Yì Jīng*[2] says: "[Enable] that which is small to come together so as to complete that which is big"; the *Shī Jīng*[3] mentions the very first birth of the people, and the *Zuǒ Zhuàn*[4] cites the fact that Shēngzǐ gave birth to Yǐngōng.

(3) The single significance of these quotes lies in the fact that from a tiny start to completion, from childhood to adulthood, human emotions manifest universally and did not wait [to be discussed until the later date of composition of] the Classics and Histories.

(4) Now the present collection of treatments is arranged by placing the treatments for women and children first, and those for husbands and the elderly afterwards. The significance of this structure is that it venerates the root.

---

1 *Dào* 道: As most readers may know, *dào* means much more than just the literal translation of "path," including notions like "method," "teachings," or even "art." You could fill a whole library with books that have been written on this key concept in classical Chinese culture and philosophy. To give interested readers just two of the major sources, see A.C. Graham, *Disputers of the Tao: Philosophical Argument in Ancient China* (Open Court, 1989) and Chad Hansen, *A Daoist Theory of Chinese Thought: A Philosophical Interpretation* (Oxford University Press, 2000).

2 *Yì Jīng* 《易經》 (Classic of Changes): This is a reference to one of the earliest classics in Chinese history. Originally a manual of divination, its significance as a philosophical or cosmological guide goes far beyond that. It is one of the five Confucian classics (*wǔjīng* 五經).

3 *Shī Jīng* 《詩經》 (Classic of Poetry): Sometimes also known as the "Book of Songs," this is another one of the Five Classics of Confucianism that dates from an extremely early time in Chinese literary history, even quoting some ritual songs from the Shāng dynasty (second millennium BCE). It is a collection of ancient songs and poetry that Sūn Sīmiǎo and his contemporaries quoted extensively to illustrate their points and to drive home moral and philosophical arguments in particular.

4 *Zuǒ Zhuàn* 《左傳》 (Chronicles of Zuǒ): This is another ancient and often-cited text that chronicles the political events in China's central states during the Spring and Autumn period (722-468 BCE).

論曰:

（一）夫生民之道，莫不以養小為大。

（二）若無於小，卒不成大。故《易》稱積小以成大；《詩》有厥初生民；《傳》云聲子生隱公。

（三）此之一義，即是從微至著，自少及長，人情共見，不待經史。

（四）故今斯方，先婦人、小兒，而後丈夫、耆老者，則是崇本之義也。

（五）然小兒氣勢微弱，醫士欲留心救療，立功瘥難。

（六）今之學者，多不存意，良由嬰兒在於襁褓之內，乳氣腥臊，醫者操行英雄，詎肯瞻視。

（七）靜而言之，可為太息者矣。

I.1 Essay

Line I.1.1, cont.

(5) Nevertheless, the force of qì[5] is still feeble in small children, and medical gentlemen[6] need to take great care to rescue and cure them and meritoriously offer their services to help them recover from serious conditions.

(6) The majority of present-day scholars fail to hold on to this intention. For this reason, when infants in swaddling clothes are concerned, surrounded by the foul stench of breast milk, how dare we look down on those doctors who carry out heroic acts?

(7) But in reference to [those doctors who] retreat/remain still,[7] all I can do is sigh deeply!

Commentary I.1 ▻ Brenda Hood

When spirit incarnates in a body, there is a process that takes place as defined later in this book as episodes of steaming and transformation. As a child is newly born, the strength of his or her qì is necessarily weak as a consequence of both the newness of the child and the fact that the child is still gathering in the resources to grow and become larger. Additionally, the new being is not yet fully able to regulate itself and so there will be swings in the relative strength or weakness of the power underlying its life processes and the processes of growth. As practitioners, we must take both of these aspects into account in the treatment of newborns and infants and not interfere overly in processes that are just beginning to come on line.

As an interesting aside to this, up until the age of about six (and perhaps even later), the qì of the child is still connected to the mother and on this level they are not fully separate. This means that clinically, in certain situations, it is possible to treat the child through the mother. This aspect of the mother - child relationship is also relevant to the discussion of intrusive upset, covered in chapter 4 of this book.

---

5 See Commentary I.1

6 *Yī shì* 醫士: I choose to translate this phrase literally here as members of the literati elite involved in medical matters.

7 *Jìng ér yán zhī* 靜而言之: The *Sūn Zhēn Rén* 《孫真人》 edition (see preface) has *tuì* 退 while modern editions have *jìng* 靜 here. Another edition from the Sòng period has *jìng yān sī zhī* 靜言思之.

（一）《小品方》云：凡人年六歲以上為小，十六歲以上為少，三十以上為壯，五十以上為老。

（二）其六歲以下，經所不載，所以乳下嬰兒有病難治者，皆為無所承據也。

（三）中古有巫妨者，立小兒《顱囟經》以占夭壽，判疾病死生，世相傳授，始有小兒方焉。

（四）逮於晉宋，江左推諸蘇家，傳習有驗，流於人間。

（五）齊有徐王者，亦有小兒方三卷。

（六）故今之學者，頗得傳授。然徐氏位望隆重，何暇留心於少小。

（七）詳其方意，不甚深細，少有可采，未為至秘。

I.1 Essay

Line I.1.2

(1) The *Xiǎo Pǐn Fāng*[1] states: All humans are considered "small" from the age of six *suì* on. From the age of sixteen *suì* on, they are considered "young." From the age of thirty *suì* on, they are considered "adult." From the age of fifty *suì* on, they are considered "old."[2]

(2) The classics record nothing on children younger than six *suì*. As a result, diseases of breastfeeding infants that are difficult to treat are nowhere recorded or attested.

(3) In mid antiquity, there was a person named Wū Fáng who wrote the *Lú Xìn Jīng*[3] for small children, to divine their premature death or longevity, and to judge whether diseases would end in life or death. Passed down to posterity, this is the first text to contain treatments for small children.

(4) Arriving at the Jìn and Liú-Sòng periods,[4] the region to the east of the Yangzi River held the various members of the Sū clan in high esteem, transmitting and collecting their experiences and passing them on among the population.

---

1 *Xiǎo Pǐn Fāng*《小品方》(Sketched-Out Formulas): Sometimes translated into English as "Digest of Formulas," this text is a brief collection of treatments that was written in the late fifth century CE by the famous physician Chén Yánzhī 陳延之.

2 *Suì* 歲: In China, human age is counted in *suì*歲, beginning from the moment of birth. A child who is four *suì* old in China is therefore three years old in English. The present phrase means literally translated "older than six *suì*," or in other words past their sixth birthday. Other early Chinese medical literature, like the *Zhū Bìng Yuán Hòu Lùn*《諸病源候論》(Discussion of the Origins and Signs of the Various Diseases) from 610 by Cháo Yuánfāng 巢元方 and the *Wài Tái Mì Yào*《外臺秘要》(Essential Secrets from a Border Official/the Palace Library) from 752 by Wáng Tāo 王燾, define youth as beginning at age eighteen and adulthood at twenty.

3 *Lú Xìn Jīng*《顱囟經》: The "Fontanel Classic" is an only partially transmitted text from either the late Zhōu or Eastern Hàn period that discusses etiologies and treatments for children so young that their fontanels have not closed yet, hence the title of the text. It is recorded in the Sòng dynasty bibliographic record as a two-volume text. In the *Zhū Bìng Yuán Hòu Lùn*, the author's name is written as Wū Fāng 巫方, which could arguably also be translated as "Treatments by Shamans."

4 *Jìn Sòng* 晉宋: These dynasties date to the third to fifth centuries BCE.

（一）《小品方》云：凡人年六歲以上為小，十六歲以上為少，三十以上為壯，五十以上為老。

（二）其六歲以下，經所不載，所以乳下嬰兒有病難治者，皆為無所承據也。

（三）中古有巫妨者，立小兒《顱囟經》以占夭壽，判疾病死生，世相傳授，始有小兒方焉。

（四）逮於晉宋，江左推諸蘇家，傳習有驗，流於人間。

（五）齊有徐王者，亦有小兒方三卷。

（六）故今之學者，頗得傳授。然徐氏位望隆重，何暇留心於少小。

（七）詳其方意，不甚深細，少有可采，未為至秘

（一）今博撰諸家及自經用有效者，以為此篇。

（二）凡百居家，皆宜達茲養小之術，則無橫夭之禍也。

I.1 Essay

Line I.1.2, cont.

(5) The state of Qí[5] had King Xú,[6] whose writings also include three volumes of treatments for small children.

(6) As a consequence, today's scholars have received a fair number of teachings. Nevertheless, Master Xú had a lofty social status, so how could he have found the leisure time to devote himself to small children?[7]

(7) When I look at the rationales behind his treatments in detail, [I realize that] they are not very profound and detailed and that there are few that are worth selecting, and none that are of consummate mystery.

Line I.1.3

(1) At present, I have made abundant selections from amongst the various masters while also including effective treatments that I have personally experienced, to compose this chapter.

(2) Each and every household should master this "art of nurturing the young," so that it will be spared the calamity of untimely death.

---

5 *Qí* 齊: Roughly equivalent with modern-day Shāndōng.

6 *Xū wáng* 徐王: This is a reference to Xú Zhīcái 徐之才, a famous doctor with high status at court from a long family lineage of physicians. He was particularly well known for his skills in compounding formulas, but also for his month-by-month instructions on nurturing the fetus during pregnancy. See my translation of Sūn Sīmiǎo's three volumes on gynecology, *Bei Ji Qian Jin Yao Fang: Essential Prescriptions worth a Thousand in Gold for Every Emergency Vol. 2-4*, pp. 101-126 for more information on this important topic. I have not been able to find any further information on the "three volumes of treatments for small children" mentioned here.

7 *Hé xiá liú xīn yú shào xiǎo* 何暇留心於少小: An alternative reading of the text, based on a changed punctuation, would be "... so how could he have found the leisure to devote himself to small children and to carefully elaborate on the intention of his formulas?"

又曰:

（一）小兒病與大人不殊，惟用藥有多少為異。

（二）其驚癇、客忤、解顱、不行等八九篇合為此卷。

（三）下痢等餘方並散在諸篇，可披而得之

I.2 Another Essay

(1) The diseases of small children are no different from those of adults. The only difference lies in the quantity of medicinals that are used.

(2) The eight or nine chapters on fright seizures[1], intrusive upset[2], separated skull[3], failure to walk[4], etc. are here combined into the present volume.

(3) Other treatments for conditions like diarrhea etc. are scattered throughout the various other volumes [of the *Bèi Jí Qiān Jīn Yào Fāng*] and can be found there.[5]

---

1 *Jīng xián* 驚癇: Fright seizures is the name of a pathocondition that is caused by an exuberance of heat in the heart and liver of young children. When this heat exuberance is compounded by fright, this condition results in derangement of the *shén* and of qì. Other key signs of fright seizures include vomiting, an abruptly alternating red and white facial complexion, and panic and disquietude, as if someone were trying to grab them. See *Zhū Bìng Yuán Hòu Lùn* vol. 45, entry 10. For more detailed descriptions and treatment strategies, see chapter three of the present book, which is dedicated to the topic of fright seizures (pp. 109-232 below).

2 *Kè wǔ* 客忤: Translated by Wiseman as "visiting hostility," this is the name of a dreadful pathocondition that is caused by a hostile intrusion of demonic qì from outside the body. The prevalence of this disease in small children in particular is related to the fact that their *shén* and qì are not yet settled and that the disease can therefore be triggered by sudden encounters with abnormal sounds or sights. Manifestations include fright and crying that will not cease, in severe cases with an abnormal facial complexion, vomiting, diarrhea, and abdominal pain, and convulsions as in fright seizures. See *Zhū Bìng Yuán Hòu Lùn* vol. 46, and chapter four of the present book, which is dedicated to the topic of intrusive upset (pp.233-292 below).

3 *Jiě lú* 解顱: Separated skull, or in other words failure of the fontanels to close at the appropriate time after birth, is the name of a pathocondition, translated as "ununited skull" by Wiseman. According to the *Zhū Bìng Yuán Hòu Lùn*, it is caused by an insufficiency of paternal essence and blood, which leads to a scarcity of prenatal kidney qì and failure to nourish the brain and marrow. See the corresponding entry in *Zhū Bìng Yuán Hòu Lùn* vol. 48, entry on "separated skull."

4 *Bù xíng* 不行: This is a reference to delayed walking, a condition that is related to kidney vacuity and soft bones due to weak prenatal endowment.

5 The following section on neonatal development is not found in the *Sūn Zhēn Rén* edition and is therefore quite possibly a later addition.

（一）凡生後六十日瞳子成，能咳笑應和人；百日任脈成，能自反覆；百八十日尻骨成，能獨坐；二百一十日掌骨成，能匍匐；三百日臏骨成，能獨立；三百六十日膝骨成，能行。

（二）此其定法。若不能依期者，必有不平之處。

I.3 Neonatal Development

(1) In all cases, sixty days after birth the pupils are completed and [babies] are able to smile and laugh and respond to people. A hundred days [after birth],[1] the Rènmài is completed and babies are able to roll over on their own. A hundred and eighty days [after birth], the bones in the buttocks are completed and babies are able to sit up on their own. Two hundred and ten days [after birth], the bones in the palm of the hand are completed and babies are able to crawl. Three hundred days [after birth], the kneecaps are completed and babies are able to stand on their own. Three hundred and sixty days [after birth], the knees are completed and babies are able to walk.

(2) This is the method to determine [the age-appropriate development of skills]. If a baby is unable to accord with this schedule, there must be some place that is out of balance.

1 Editorial note: Another edition of the text has a hundred and fifty days here.

（一）凡兒生三十二日一變，六十四日再變，變且蒸；九十六日三變，一百二十八日四變，變且蒸；一百六十日五變，一百九十二日六變，變且蒸；二百二十四日七變，二百五十六日八變，變且蒸；二百八十八日九變，三百二十日十變，變且蒸。

（二）積三百二十日小蒸畢後，六十四日大蒸，蒸後六十四日複大蒸，蒸後一百二十八日複大蒸。

（三）凡小兒，自生三十二日一變，再變為一蒸。

（四）凡十變而五小蒸，又三大蒸，積五百七十六日，大小蒸都畢，乃成人。

（五）小兒所以變蒸者，是榮其血脈，改其五臟，故一變竟輒覺情態有異。

I.4 Transformations And Steamings[1]

Line I.4.1

(1) In all cases, babies undergo a first transformation on the 32nd day after birth and a second transformation on the 64th day, which is a combination of transforming and steaming.[2] The third transformation occurs on the 96th day and the fourth transformation on the 128th day, which is again a combination of transforming and steaming. The fifth transformation occurs on the 160th day and the sixth transformation on the 192nd day, which is again a combination of transforming and steaming. The seventh transformation occurs on the 224th day and the eighth transformation on the 256th day, which is again a combination of transforming and steaming. The ninth transformation occurs on the 288th day and the tenth transformation on the 320th day, which is again a combination of transforming steaming.

(2) After the minor steaming that occurs when the full 320 days are completed, there is a major steaming 64 days later and then, an additional 64 days after that steaming, yet another major steaming, and then, after another 128 days, yet another major steaming.

(3) In all cases, babies undergo a first transformation 32 days after birth, and then a second transformation, which constitutes the first steaming.

(4) In all cases, there are ten transformations and five minor steamings, and then three major steamings, which take place within a total of 576 days [after birth]. When the major and minor steamings are all finished, [the baby] has become a human being.

(5) The reason why babies pass through these transformations and steamings is so as to make their blood and vessels thrive and alter their five *zàng* organs. For this reason, as soon as the first transformation is finished, you can sense a difference in their condition right away.

---

1 See Commentary I.2 on p. 16 below.

2 According to the *Zhū Bìng Yuán Hòu Lùn* (vol. 45, entry 2), "transformations and steamings" (*biàn zhēng* 變蒸) signify the growth of blood and qì. *Biàn* 變 ("transformation") refers to the ascent of qì, while *zhēng* 蒸 ("steaming") refers to the presence of heat in the body. The key sign by which we differentiate transformations and steamings from conditions of heat or cold damage is that while the body is hot, the ears and buttocks are cold.

（一）其變蒸之候，變者上氣，蒸者體熱。

（二）變蒸有輕重，其輕者，體熱而微驚，耳冷尻冷，上唇頭白泡起，如魚目珠子，微汗出；其重者，體壯熱而脈亂，或汗或不汗，不欲食，食輒吐哯，目白睛微赤，黑睛微白。

（三）又云：目白者重，赤黑者微。

（四）變蒸畢，目睛明矣，此其証也。

Commentary I.2 ▻ Brenda Hood

Transformations and steamings as described in this text seem to point to the idea that they are part of the normal process of incarnating and becoming a human being. Given this, I think it makes an interesting contrast to the modern obsession with reducing fever in infants.

According to Chinese medicine theory, infants are pure yáng transforming into a yīn body. The classical description says that this is the reason that small children run everywhere. The Moon is the ultimate reference to yīn so this statement may be a way of saying that transformations and steamings are part of the process of spirit/consciousness incarnating into human form.

I.4 Transformations And Steamings

Line I.4.2

(1) The signs for transformations and steamings are as follows: Transformation refers to the ascent of qì, and steaming refers to heat in the body.

(2) Transformations and steamings can be mild or intense.[1] If they are mild, we see heat in the body with mild fright, cold ears and buttocks, white blisters breaking out on the upper lip and head that resemble fish eyes or pearls, and slight sweating. If they are serious, we see vigorous heat in the body accompanied by a disordered pulse, whether with sweating or without sweating, a lack of appetite, vomiting right after nursing, and slight redness in the white of the eye and slight whiteness in the black of the eyes.

(3) It is also said that whiteness of the eyes signifies intense [conditions], while redness or blackness signifies mild ones.

(4) When the transformations and steamings are finished, the eyeballs become bright! This is the evidence [that this stage is over].

1 Unfortunately, the text provides no explanations for why, how, and when this series of normal developmental changes might become pathological. My best guess is that the baby's overall state of health at the specific points in time, compounded perhaps by particularly attentive infant care by the mother or other caregivers, may allow him or her to weather these stages with more or less pronounced symptoms. In either case, the key point of this passage appears to be that it is crucial for the family to prepare for and recognize these symptoms as normal expressions of neonatal development, rather than as manifestations of a pathology that would be in need of treatment.

（一）單變小微，兼蒸小劇。

（二）凡蒸平者，五日而衰，遠者十日而衰。

（三）先期五日，後之五日，為十日之中，熱乃除耳。

（四）兒生三十二日一變，二十九日先期而熱，便治之如法，至三十六七日蒸乃畢耳。

（五）恐不解了，故重說之。

I.4 Transformations And Steamings

Line I.4.3

(1) Transformations on their own are minor and mild, but in combination with steaming [become] mildly acute.

(2) In all cases, steamings abate in five days when they are normal but abate in ten days when they are more far-reaching.

(3) With five days prior to the time [of steaming] and five days afterwards, [the numbers given above][1] fall in the middle of these ten days. After that, the heat should be expelled.

(4) For the first transformation, which takes place 32 days after the baby's birth, the heat will begin prior to this around the 29th day. If you handle this state in accordance with this rule, when the 36th or 37th day arrives, the steaming will finish[2] and that's all.

(5) Since I fear that you did not understand this [initially], I have explained it again.

---

1 Specifically, this refers to days 64, 128, 192, 256, etc. after birth, for the first, second, third, fourth, etc. steamings. Alternately, this list could also include the days given for transformations that occur without steamings, but this would slightly contradict the following statement that gives the range of generalized heat for simple transformations as five days, not ten.

2 It appears slightly contradictory that this line, a discussion of the first transformation at day 32 after birth, which is supposed to be only a transformation but not in combination with steaming, mentions the end of steaming around day 36 or 37. My best guess is that even plain transformations involve a certain degree of heat effusion and that "steaming" is used in this line to refer more generally to the state of the body resulting from the ascent of heat. This line of reasoning is corroborated by line I.5.1 on p. 25 below, which states that, "transformation means generalized heat."

（一）且變蒸之時，不欲驚動，勿令旁多人。

（二）兒變蒸或早或晚，不如法者多。

（三）又初變之時，或熱甚者，違日數不歇，審計變蒸之日，當其時有熱微驚，慎不可治及灸刺，但和視之。

（四）若良久熱不可已，少與紫丸微下，熱歇便止。

I.4 Transformations And Steamings

Line I.4.4

(1) In addition, at the time of transformations and steamings, do not expose [babies] to fright or [too much] activity. Do not allow a lot of people by their side.

(2) It is quite common that children's transformations and steamings occur either early or late and not according to the rule [given above].[1]

(3) Furthermore, at the time of the onset of transformations, there are some cases where the heat is severe and fails to subside, in violation of the number of days. Calculate the days of transformations and steamings precisely, [since these are] the right times when you should see heat and mild fright. Beware: You must not treat [with medications] or apply moxibustion or acupuncture! Only keep them company and observe them.

(4) If it has been a good long while and you are unable to stop the heat, give a little bit of Zǐ Wán[2] to induce a mild downward action.[3] The heat will subside and then stop.

---

1 *Bù rú fǎ zhě duō* 不如法者多: This statement is interesting, but from a clinical perspective not surprising. While it appears to be a direct contradiction to the emphatic use of *fán* 凡 ("in all cases") in numerous lines above, but especially in line I.4.1 on p. 15, where the author claims that transformations and steamings always occur on specific days after the birth, I see it simply as a needed correction. As any medical practitioner knows, human bodies differ and don't follow strict rules. To me, this line is a welcome sign for the practical orientation of Sūn Sīmiǎo's writing.

2 Zǐ Wán 紫丸: Literally, "Purple Pill." The formula is found following this essay, on pp. 33-35 below.

3 *Wēi xià* 微下: For the sake of clarity over elegance, I have chosen to preserve the literal meaning of *xià* 下 ("down," so in the verbal sense "to bring down"). Nevertheless, the use of the term here (as in most descriptions of intended formula actions below) clearly implies the induction of a bowel movement, which is the intended direct action of the present formula. Wiseman translates *xià* 下 across the board as "precipitation," but I prefer the more literal and broader, if less elegant, translation as "downward action" or "bringing down," because that best conveys the meaning of the character without implying the conversion from a gaseous to a liquid state. Alternatively, the phrase can here be read as "a mild reduction [in heat]," which would certainly make perfect sense as well.

（一）若於變蒸之中，加以時行溫病，或非變蒸時而得時行者，其診皆相似，惟耳及尻通熱，口上無白泡耳。

（二）當先服黑散以發其汗，汗出，溫粉粉之，熱當歇，便就瘥。

（三）若猶不都除，乃與紫丸下之。

（四）兒變蒸時，若有寒加之，即寒熱交爭，腹腰夭糺，啼不止者，熨之則愈也。

（五）變蒸與溫壯傷寒相似，若非變蒸，身熱，耳熱，尻亦熱，此乃為他病，可作餘治。

（六）審是變蒸，不得為餘治也。

I.4 Transformations And Steamings

Line I.4.5

(1) If in the middle of a transformation or steaming the condition is further complicated by a seasonal warm disease, or if it is not the time for a transformation or steaming and [the baby] has [only] contracted a seasonal disease, the diagnosis is similar in both of these cases, namely simply the presence of heat penetrating through to the ears and buttocks and the absence of white blisters above the mouth.

(2) [For such conditions,] first administer Hēi Sǎn[1] to promote sweating. When the sweat is coming out, sprinkle warm rice flour[2] on [the baby's body] and the heat should subside. This indicates recovery.

(3) If it is still not all eliminated, in that case give Zǐ Wán to bring down [the pathological heat].[3]

(4) At the times of a child's transformations and steamings, if the condition is further complicated by cold, the cold and heat struggle with each other. This causes [the patient] to bend and twist at the abdomen and lumbus and to cry incessantly. In such cases, treat by applying a hot compress,[4] which will result in recovery.

(5) Transformations and steamings are similar to severe warmth seen in cold damage. If it is not a case of a transformation or steaming, you will see generalized heat with heat in the ears and also in the buttocks. This signifies that it is a different condition, which you may manage with additional treatment.

(6) If you have identified the condition as a transformation or steaming, you may not administer additional treatment.

---

1 Hēi Sǎn 黑散: Literally, "Black Powder." The formula is found following this essay, on pp. 42-43 below.

2 *Wēn fěn fěn zhī* 温粉粉之: It is unclear to me whether this refers to the specific name of a different formula for "Warm Powder" or simply to heated rice flour. I have been unable to find a formula with the name Wēn Fěn 温粉.

3 *Xià zhī* 下之: Regardless of how we interpret *xià* 下, here it means to eliminate the heat by inducing a bowel movement.

4 *Yùn zhī* 熨之: Instructions for this hot compress method are found in the following chapter, namely the treatment for Zhì Fěn Xù Yùn 炙粉絮熨 (lit., "Toasted Powder Cotton Compress"). See pp. 65-67 below.

（一）凡兒生三十二日始變，變者，身熱也。

（二）至六十四日再變，變且蒸，其狀臥端正也。

（三）至九十六日三變，定者，候丹孔出而泄。

（四）至一百二十八日四變，變且蒸，以能咳笑也。

（五）至一百六十日五變，以成機關也。

（六）至一百九十二日六變，變且蒸，五機成也。

（七）至二百二十四日七變，以能匍匐也。

（八）至二百五十六日八變，變且蒸，以知欲學語也。

（九）至二百八十八日九變，以亭亭然也。

I.5 Another Method[1]

Line I.5.1

(1) In all cases, the first transformation occurs 32 days after the baby is born. Transformation [means] generalized heat.

(2) Arriving at the 64th day, there is another transformation, which is a combination of transformation and steaming. The manifestation of this stage is that the baby is lying prone but [wanting to] straighten out.[2]

1 This essay seems to be a quotation from another source, repeating much of the previous information but fleshing it out by combining it with other markers of neonatal development. As such, it can serve as evidence for the composite nature of Sūn Sīmiǎo's writings. It is, however, found not only in the editions of the *Qiān Jīn Fāng* that postdate the Sòng revisions but already in the *Sūn Zhēn Rén* edition and was therefore most likely a part of the original text. In that version, it is interestingly enough preceded by the title, *Xiǎo Ér Biàn Zhēng Zhuàng* 小兒變蒸狀, "The Manifestation of Transformations and Steamings in Neonates."

2 *Qí zhuàng wò duān zhèng yě* 其狀臥端正也: This might be a reference to the baby's ability to lift the head and straighten out the body. Alternately, *wò* 臥 also has the meaning "to crouch," in the sense of crouching animals or birds. According to the *Shuō Wén Jiě Zì*《說文解字》("Explaining Simple Characters and Analyzing Compound Characters"), *wò* is identical in meaning to *xiū* 休 ("to rest") but is derived pictographically from the combination of *rén* 人 ("human") and *chén* 臣 ("servant"), meaning a person prostrating him- or herself in front of a lord. My reading of the present line is based on the *Sūn Zhēn Rén* edition, which has *wò yù duān zhèng* 臥欲端正. The *Shuō Wén Jiě Zì* is one of the oldest Chinese dictionaries that was compiled by Xǔ Shèn 許慎 in the late Hàn period. It gives synonyms and exemplary usages, explains the structure of characters, and, where applicable, discusses the etymology. Hence it offers an insider's perspective on the early meaning of characters and can often be helpful when trying to understand obscure passages. Yet another possible interpretation is to read *zhèng* 正 not as "straighten out" but literally as "upright," or in other words in the sense that the baby has a desire to be more vertical.

(一) 凡兒生三十二日始變，變者，身熱也。

(二) 至六十四日再變，變且蒸，其狀臥端正也。

(三) 至九十六日三變，定者，候丹孔出而泄。

(四) 至一百二十八日四變，變且蒸，以能咳笑也。

(五) 至一百六十日五變，以成機關也。

(六) 至一百九十二日六變，變且蒸，五機成也。

(七) 至二百二十四日七變，以能匍匐也。

(八) 至二百五十六日八變，變且蒸，以知欲學語也。

(九) 至二百八十八日九變，以亭亭然也。

I.5 Another Method

Line I.5.1, cont.

(3) Arriving at the third transformation on the 96th day, the sign to determine [this developmental stage] is that something is exiting and draining from the cinnabar hole.[3]

(4) Arriving at the fourth transformation on the 128th day, which is a combination of transformation and steaming, the baby is consequently able to cough and laugh.

(5) Arriving at the fifth transformation on the 160th day, consequently the mechanisms for opening and closing are completed.[4]

---

3 *Hòu dān kǒng chū ér xiè* 候丹孔出而泄: The medical historian Yi-Li Wu has pointed out that the hundredth day is historically the time for special ceremonies that formally incorporate the neonate into the family because the baby has finally passed through the most vulnerable period. The concept of *dān* 丹, which literally means "cinnabar," is multi-layered and definitely in need of a lengthier explanation than the limitations of this book allow. Park Yung-hwan explains that the character is a combination of 井 (well) and 石 (stone), meaning " a well for digging up stones," in other words a well that was dug to procure multi-colored stones and most notably the precious red stone cinnabar. In the context of pediatrics, *dān* is linked to eruptions of *tāi dú* 胎毒 ("fetal poison"), which in later times is believed to reside in the *mìng mén* 命門(Life Gate), a mysterious area in the body that is sometimes conflated with the *dān tiān* 丹田 (Cinnabar Field). The *Wài Kē Qǐ Xuán* 《外科啟玄》("Opening the Mysteries of External Medicine"), a text composed in 1602 by Shēn Gǒngchén 申拱辰, includes ten illustrations of a pediatric disease called *dān* (cinnabar), which is explained as various patterns of *tāi dú* (fetal poison) erupting on the body. In the explanation of cinnabar as a skin disease in adults, the same text equates *dān* with *chì* 赤("red") and explains that the disease looks like the skin has been painted or dotted with red paint or ink. Yi-Li Wu therefore suggests that the transformation of the 96th day has to do with something that is draining out from the *dān* orifice, which may be the idea of a fetal poison that finally leaves the body and can no longer threaten the health of the infant. In a more clinical orientation, Arnaud Versluys suggests a definition as "noxious (contagious?) illness with cinnabar red clinical signs of mostly dermatological or surgical nature, due to a damp heat etiology." I am much indebted to the scholars and practitioners mentioned above for their insights into this subject.

4 *Jī guān* 機關: I read this expression fairly literally as the major structural junctures (i.e., the locations and entities in charge of opening and closing) of the body. *Guān* can also refer more specifically to the joints, as in the common modern compound *guān jié* 關節.

（一）凡兒生三十二日始變，變者，身熱也。

（二）至六十四日再變，變且蒸，其狀臥端正也。

（三）至九十六日三變，定者，候丹孔出而泄。

（四）至一百二十八日四變，變且蒸，以能咳笑也。

（五）至一百六十日五變，以成機關也。

（六）至一百九十二日六變，變且蒸，五機成也。

（七）至二百二十四日七變，以能匍匐也。

（八）至二百五十六日八變，變且蒸，以知欲學語也。

（九）至二百八十八日九變，以亭亭然也。

I.5 Another Method

Line I.5.1, cont.
(6) Arriving at the sixth transformation on the 192nd day, which is a combination of transformation and steaming, the five mechanisms[5] are completed.

(7) Arriving at the seventh transformation on the 224th day, [the child] is consequently able to crawl.

(8) Arriving at the eighth transformation on the 256th day, which is a combination of transformation and steaming, [the child] consequently has awareness of its desire to learn how to speak.

(9) Arriving at the ninth transformation on the 288th day, [the child] is consequently able to stand erect.

---

5 *Wǔ jī* 五機: Some editions have *jī* 機 here, some have *zàng* 臟 (zàng organs/ viscera). The *Sūn Zhēn Rén* edition has *bìn gǔ* 髕骨 ("kneecaps"). *Jī* is explained as originally referring to the trigger mechanism for releasing arrows from a bow or a loom for spinning, and then by extension to any triggering mechanism. I have kept my translation intentionally vague so that readers may make up their own mind on what this term means here. Interpreting it as *zàng* organs is definitely a good option, especially since there are five of them, but narrows the meaning down too much for my taste. It is equally possible that the term refers to some sort of mechanisms associated with the five dynamic movements (*wǔ xíng* 五行).

（一）凡小兒生至二百八十八日，九變四蒸也。

（二）當其變之日，慎不可妄治之，則加其疾。

（三）變且蒸者，是兒送迎月也。

（四）蒸者，甚熱而脈亂，汗出是也，近者五日歇，遠者八九日歇也。

（五）當是蒸上，不可灸刺妄治之也。

I.5 Another Method

Line I.5.2

(1) Whenever newborns have reached the 288th day after birth, [there should have been] nine transformations and four steamings.

(2) On the days of any steamings, beware! You may not recklessly treat it, or you will only add to the [child's] illness.

(3) Transformations in combination with steamings mean that the child is sending off and welcoming the moon.[1]

(4) Steaming is precisely [characterized by] severe heat with chaos in the vessels and sweating. When it is limited, it subsides in five days. When it is extensive, it subsides in eight or nine days.

(5) During any of these steamings, you may not apply moxibustion or acupuncture, or recklessly treat it [with medicinals].

---

1 The *Sūn Zhēn Rén* edition has *nì yíng* 逆迎 instead of *sòng yíng* 送迎. This could be interpreted as "...the baby is rebelling against welcoming the moon." The meaning of either version is unclear to me. I am indebted to Dr. Brenda Hood for pointing out that babies are pure *yáng* transforming into a *yīn* body. Given the fact that the moon is the ultimate reference to *yīn*, this may be a way of saying that transformations and steamings are part of the process by which Spirit incarnates into human flesh..

紫丸

治小兒變蒸，發熱不解，並挾傷寒溫壯，汗後熱不歇，及腹中有痰癖，哺乳不進，乳則吐哯 食癇，先寒後熱者方。

代赭	一兩
赤石脂	一兩
巴豆	三十枚
杏仁	五十枚

（一）上四味，末之。巴豆、杏仁別研為膏，相和，更擣二千杵，當自相得。若硬，入少蜜同擣之，密器中收。

（二）三十日兒服如麻子一丸，與少乳汁令下。食頃後，與少乳勿令多。至日中當小下，熱除。

（三）若未全除，明旦更與一丸。

（四）百日兒服如小豆一丸，以此準量增減。

（五）夏月多熱，喜令發疹，二三十日輒一服佳。

（六）紫丸無所不療，雖下不虛人。

I.6 Zǐ Wán (Purple Pill)

Indications

A formula to treat transformations and steamings in young children with heat effusion that fails to resolve, compounded by vigorous warmth from cold damage, heat that does not subside after sweating, as well as the presence of phlegm aggregations[1] in the abdomen, inability to ingest breast milk or other foods,vomiting upon nursing, food seizures,[2] and first [aversion to] cold and then heat [effusion].

Ingredients

dàizhě	1 *liǎng*
chìshízhī	1 *liǎng*
bādòu	30 pieces
xìngrén	50 pieces

Preparation

(1) Pulverize the four ingredients above. [First] grind the *bādòu* and *xìngrén* separately into a paste, then mix everything together. Pound it another 2000 times with a pestle until it is all thoroughly blended. If it is [too] stiff, add a little honey and pound it in. Store in a tightly sealed jar.

---

1 *Tán pǐ* 痰癖: Phlegm aggregations are explained in the *Zhū Bìng Yuán Hòu Lùn* as a condition that is "caused by drinking water but failing to disperse it. When this water encounters cold or heat qì in the area of the chest, they struggle with each other, as the result of which the water becomes deep-lying and stagnant and forms phlegm. As the phlegm becomes chronic and collects, it moves into the rib-sides and causes periodic pain there." According to Gé Hóng 葛洪 in the *Bào Pǔ Zǐ*《抱朴子》(chapter on *Jī Yán* 機言), "Excessive eating results in binding accumulations and gatherings; excessive drinking results in the formation of phlegm aggregations." The "Master who Embraces Simplicity," which is the literal translation of *Bào Pǔ Zǐ*, is a philosophical text, primarily Daoist in orientation, that dates from the early fourth century CE.

2 *Shí xián* 食癇: This symptom is explained in volume 85 of the *Tài Píng Shèng Huì Fāng*《太平聖惠方》as a condition that is caused by immoderate consumption of breast milk or by illness in the spleen and stomach. Either of these conditions cause the milk to stagnate, transform into phlegm, and engender heat, which ascends to harass the spirit. It manifests with vomiting of acid rotten liquid, convulsions in the extremities, and upward-staring eyes. The *Tài Píng Shèng Huì Fāng* ("Sagely Grace Formulary from the Taìpíng Era") is an encyclopedic collection of treatments that was compiled on imperial orders by the Sòng dynasty under the leadership of Wáng Huáiyǐn 王懷隱. See also *Zhū Bìng Yuán Hòu Lùn*, vol. 45, entry on *xián* 癇 "seizures."

紫丸

治小兒變蒸，發熱不解，並挾傷寒溫壯，汗後熱不歇，及腹中有痰癖，哺乳不進，乳則吐哯 食癇，先寒後熱者方。

代赭	一兩
赤石脂	一兩
巴豆	三十枚
杏仁	五十枚

（一）上四味，末之。巴豆、杏仁別研為膏，相和，更擣二千杵，當自相得。若硬，入少蜜同擣之，密器中收。

（二）三十日兒服如麻子一丸，與少乳汁令下。食頃後，與少乳勿令多。至日中當小下，熱除。

（三）若未全除，明旦更與一丸。

（四）百日兒服如小豆一丸，以此準量增減。

（五）夏月多熱，喜令發疹，二三十日輒一服佳。

（六）紫丸無所不療，雖下不虛人。

I.6 Zǐ Wán (Purple Pill)

Preparation, cont.

(2) For a 30-day-old child, administer one pill the size of a hemp seed. Give it with a little breast milk to make it go down. After about the time it takes to eat a meal, again give a small amount of breast milk, but not a lot. Wait until mid-day and there should be a small downward movement.[3] This is the heat being eliminated.

(3) If [the heat] is not eliminated completely [by this first treatment], give another pill on the next morning.

(4) For a 100-day-old child, administer one pill the size of an aduki bean. Using this as a norm, increase or decrease [the dosage].

(5) During the summer months when there is a profusion of heat [in the outside environment], [young children] have a tendency to develop rashes. [Under these circumstances], it is excellent to administer one dose every 20 or 30 days.

(6) There is nothing that Zǐ Wán does not cure. In spite of its down-draining effect, it does not make the person vacuous.

---

3 In the present context, I am quite certain that the descending action of xià 下 here refers to the intended medicinal action of inducing a bowel movement to eliminate the disease-causing agent. The effect of the medicinal ingredients also confirms this interpretation.

紫丸《千金要方衍義》

（一）初生變蒸雖所禀不足，而於不足之中必有痰癖內結，所以蒸發寒熱。

（二）紫丸一方藥品頗峻，而用法最緩。

（三）設慮其峻而因循，不即下手，即將來乳哺，日蘊為痰，有增無減，為驚為癇，靡不由此。

（四）方以石脂溫養心脾，代赭除腹中邪氣，杏仁下氣散寒熱，雖用巴豆蕩練臟腑，以二石護持中土，故叮嚀致再，服之無傷。

Zǐ Wán (Purple Pill) *Yǎn Yì* (Expanded Meaning)

(1) Regarding transformations and steamings in newborns, while constitutional insufficiency does play a role, this insufficiency must be compounded by phlegm aggregations binding internally in order for the steamings to erupt as chills and fevers.

(2) The medicinal ingredients in the formula for Zǐ Wán are rather drastic, and it must be used with extreme moderation.[1]

(3) [Nevertheless,] if you consider this drastic nature and hence delay its use instead of immediately taking action, as a result when the baby nurses or feeds in the future, [the food] will smolder day after day [in the baby's digestive system] and turn into phlegm, ever increasing and never decreasing. This situation will cause fright and seizures. [These conditions] are invariably caused by this.[2]

(4) The formula uses *chìshízhī* to warm and nourish the heart and spleen, *dàizhě* to eliminate the evil qì from inside the abdomen, and *xìngrén* to bring the qì down and dissipate cold and heat. Even though it uses *bādòu* to flush out and scour the *zàng* and *fǔ* organs, it takes advantage of the two mineral substances[3] to protect and sustain center earth. Therefore I reiterate yet again: Administering [this formula properly] does not cause any damage.

---

1 *Yòng fǎ zuì huǎn* 用法最緩: In other words, you must exercise extreme caution to administer age-appropriate dosages to small children. An alternative reading could be "...and yet its usage is extremely moderate," meaning that its effect is not as dramatic as the strong ingredients might suggest, or in other words actually surprisingly safe to use. This interpretation does not make much clinical sense in this context, however, namely a discussion of the effect of a strongly down-draining formula on newborn babies.

2 *Mí bù yóu cǐ* 靡不由此: Or in other words, by this failure to address steaming in conjunction with phlegm aggregations by means of drastic medical intervention.

3 *Èr shí* 二石: Here, clearly a reference to the two mineral ingredients *chìshízhī* and *dàizhě*.

紫丸《千金要方衍義》

（一）允為防微杜漸之的方，瀉中寓補之捷法也。

（二）一其後驚癇門論中有云：四味紫丸逐癖飲最良，去病速而不虛人。赤丸瘥駃，病重者當用之。

（三）林億云：方中並無赤丸，次後癖結脹滿篇中雙紫丸內有朱砂，色當赤，又力緊於紫丸，疑此即赤丸也。

（四）按《金匱》腹滿寒疝宿食篇中有赤丸，方用茯苓、半夏、烏頭、細辛，蜜丸，真朱為色，

（五）《千金》不用細辛作人參，專治寒氣厥逆，以中有半夏、烏頭之反激，且有真朱之蕩癖，未嘗不散寒積也。

Zǐ Wán (Purple Pill) *Yǎn Yì* (Expanded Meaning)

(1) It is the perfect formula for nipping this condition in the bud.[1] It is also a prompt method for draining the center while supplementing.

(2) The essay in the chapter on "Fright Seizures" below[2] contains the following quotation: "Sì Wèi Zǐ Wán is outstanding for expelling aggregations and rheum, by removing the illness speedily but without causing vacuity in the person. Chì Wán makes for a speedy recovery. Use it for conditions that are critical."

(3) Lín Yì[3] states: "Among the formulas [in the referenced chapter], however, there is no entry on Chì Wán. But later on [in the *Qiān Jīn Fāng*] in the chapter on 'Aggregations, Bindings, Distention and Fullness,' the formula for Shuāng Zǐ Wán contains *zhūshā*, so its color must be red. Moreover, its strength is also more urgent than Zǐ Wán. So I wonder whether the Chì Wán mentioned here does not refer to that formula.

1 Literally translated, *fáng wēi dù jiàn* 防微杜漸 means to take preventative measures to address something tiny and thereby stop its gradual growth [and development into a much bigger problem].

2 This essay is found in section III.1 in chapter 2 below. The two formulas mentioned in this line, namely Sì Wèi Zǐ Wán and Chì Wán are found on pp. 119-121.

3 Lín Yì 林億 was a famous physician of the Sòng period who was instrumental in the imperially sponsored publication of revised and annotated editions -- and therefore preservation -- of all the early classics that have been transmitted to the present. The extent to which Lín Yì and his team altered the source texts is still subject to vigorous debate. The present quotation by Lín Yì obviously is not a response to the line in the *Yǎn Yì*, but to a different reference to Chì Wán in the chapter below on fright seizures.

紫丸《千金要方衍義》

（一）允為防微杜漸之的方，瀉中寓補之捷法也。

（二）一其後驚癇門論中有云：四味紫丸逐癖飲最良，去病速而不虛人。赤丸瘥駃，病重者當用之。

（三）林億云：方中並無赤丸，次後癖結脹滿篇中雙紫丸內有朱砂，色當赤，又力緊於紫丸，疑此即赤丸也。

（四）按《金匱》腹滿寒疝宿食篇中有赤丸，方用茯苓、半夏、烏頭、細辛，蜜丸，真朱為色，

（五）《千金》不用細辛作人參，專治寒氣厥逆，以中有半夏、烏頭之反激，且有真朱之蕩癖，未嘗不散寒積也。

Zǐ Wán (Purple Pill) *Yǎn Yì* (Expanded Meaning), cont.

(4) The Jīn Guì Yào Lüè[4] contains a formula for Chì Wán in the chapter on "Abdominal Fullness, Cold Mounting, and Abiding Food." This formula uses *fúlíng, bànxià, wūtóu,* and *xìxīn* to make honey pills, and the *zhēnzhū*[5] is responsible for the color.

(5) The *Qiān Jīn Fāng* does not use *xìxīn*, but uses *rénshēn* instead, which specifically treats reverse flow of cold qì. In the formula [for Zǐ Wán above], we find *bànxià* and *wūtóu* included for their ability to turn around [incorrect flow] and to stimulate, as well as *zhēnzhū* for its ability to flush out aggregations. This will never fail to dissipate cold accumulations.

---

4 *Jīn Guì Yào Lüè* 《金匱要略》: The "Essentials from the Golden Cabinet" is one of the most important formula texts ever written in Chinese history. Like its celebrated counterpart, the *Shāng Hán Lùn* 《傷寒論》 ("Discussion of Cold Damage"), it was composed in the Hàn period by the outstanding physician Zhāng Zhòngjǐng 張仲景. For an annotated translation of the first half of this important text, see Sabine Wilms, transl., *Formulas from the Golden Cabinet with Songs, vols. I-III* (The Chinese Medicine Database, 2010).

5 *Zhēn zhū* 真朱: Literally translated "true crimson," this is a synonym for *zhūshā* 硃砂 (cinnabar) and does not mean "pearl" here (usually written as 珍珠, but pronounced identically as *zhēnzhū*).

黑散

治小兒變蒸中挾時行溫病，或非變蒸時而得時行者方。

麻黄	半兩
大黄	六銖
杏仁	半兩

（一）上三味，先搗麻黄、大黄為散，別研杏仁如脂，乃細細納散，又搗令調和，納密器中。

（二）一月兒服小豆大一枚，以乳汁和服，抱令得汗，汗出，溫粉粉之。勿使見風。

（三）百日兒服如棗核，以兒大小量之。

I.7 Hēi Săn (Black Powder)

Indications

A formula for small children that treats transformations and steamings complicated by seasonal warm disease, or seasonally contracted diseases that do not fall within the time of transformations and steamings.

Ingredients

máhuáng	0.5 *liăng*
dàhuáng	6 *zhū*
xìngrén	0.5 *liăng*

Preparation

(1) Of the three ingredients above, first pound the *máhuáng* and *dàhuáng* into powder. Separately grind the *xìngrén* until it resembles lard and then little by little add it to the powdered [ingredients]. Pound it again until [everything is] evenly blended and fill it and seal it in a jar.

(2) For a one-month-old child, administer a single piece the size of an aduki bean. Administer it mixed into breast milk and then wrap the child to induce sweating. When the sweat is coming out, sprinkle warm rice flour[1] [on the child]. Do not allow [the patient] to be exposed to wind.

(3) For a 100-day-old child, administer a pill the size of a jujube pit. Measure [the medicine] in accordance with the child's age.

---

1 See line I.4.5, note 2 on p. 23 above.

黑散《千金要方衍義》

（一）於變蒸之中，復挾時行邪氣，非急為開提中外，何以保全萬一。

（二）方中大黃蕩滌內結，即用麻黃開發表邪，杏仁疏利逆氣。

（三）蓋大黃原有安和五臟之功，麻黃兼有破除癥堅之力，杏仁交通中外，乃麻黃湯之變方，守真通聖雙解，從此悟出。

Hēi Sǎn (Black Powder) *Yǎn Yì* (Expanded Meaning)

(1) When in the midst of transformations or steamings [a condition] is additionally complicated by seasonal evil qì, if you do not urgently open up the center to the outside, how could you keep even a single one out of ten thousand [patients] safe?

(2) In the formula, *dàhuáng* flushes out internal bindings. The formula also uses *máhuáng* to open up and effuse exterior evil, and *xìngrén* to course and disinhibit counterflow qì.

(3) Now, *dàhuáng* originally has the effect of quieting and harmonizing the five *zàng* organs, *máhuáng* also has the effect of breaking up and eliminating concretions and hardenings, and *xìngrén* opens up communication between the center and the outside. Thus [this formula] is a variation on Máhuáng Tāng. Guarding the true [qì], this formula penetrates the sagely [method of] dual resolution. From this perspective, I have come to realize this insight.

擇乳母法

（一）凡乳母者，其血氣為乳汁也。

（二）五情善惡，悉是血氣所生也。

（三）其乳兒者，皆宜慎於喜怒。

（四）夫乳母形色所宜，其候甚多，不可求備。

（五）但取不胡臭、瘻瘻、氣嗽、瘑疥、痴瘻、白禿、癧瘍、沈唇、耳聾、齆鼻、癲癇，無此等疾者，便可飲兒也。

（六）師見其故灸瘢，便知其先疾之源也。

I.8 Method For Selecting A Wet Nurse

(1) In all cases, [note that] when selecting a wet nurse, her blood and qì are what make the breast milk.

(2) The five emotions and likes and aversions are precisely what her blood and qì are engendered from.

(3) When she is nursing a child, she must beware of any joy and anger.

(4) Now regarding the appearance and complexion of a wet nurse, the signs to determine her suitability are extremely numerous, and it is impossible to seek complete perfection.

擇乳母法

（一）凡乳母者，其血氣為乳汁也。

（二）五情善惡，悉是血氣所生也。

（三）其乳兒者，皆宜慎於喜怒。

（四）夫乳母形色所宜，其候甚多，不可求備。

（五）但取不胡臭、瘿瘻、氣嗽、瘑疥、痴癃、白禿、癧瘍、沈唇、耳聾、齆鼻、癲癇，無此等疾者，便可飲兒也。

（六）師見其故灸瘢，便知其先疾之源也。

Commentary I.3 ▹ Brenda Hood

In classical times, much of the moxibustion therapy carried out left scars. This was done deliberately and was thought to increase the efficacy of the treatment. With reference to using moxa on infants, I cannot say if they still practiced scarification moxa or not, though it is possible that they did. I base this on the warning by Sūn Sīmiǎo translated in note 2 of II.6.2 on page 71 of this text of the "cruel pain" negatively affecting the infant.

I.8 Method For Selecting A Wet Nurse

(5) Nevertheless, select one without strong body odor, goiters or fistulas, coughing, *guā* sores[1] and scaly skin, a feeble mind or dribbling urinary block, white hair or baldness, scrofula[2], tight lips[3], deafness, nasal congestion, and seizures. If the candidate is free of all of these problems, then you can let her nurse the child.

(6) A teacher once said[4] that you can know the origin of previous illnesses by looking at a person's old moxibustion scars.[5,6]

1 *Guā* 瘑: According to the *Zhū Bìng Yuán Hòu Lùn* (vol. 35), this is a condition caused by emptiness in the interstices and by wind and dampness breaking up blood and qì and gathering internally. The condition manifests with markings that resemble young evodia seeds and erupt on the hands and feet. They are itchy and painful and when scratched, break and ooze a yellow fluid that spreads and forms sores.

2 *Lì yáng* 癧瘍: According to the *Zhū Bìng Yuán Hòu Lùn* (vol. 31), scrofula is a condition caused by wind evil striking the skin and causing disharmony of blood and qì. It is marked by interconnected round white or dark spots on the side of the neck, front of the chest, and below the armpits. They are not necessarily painful or itchy.

3 *Chén chún* 沈唇 is the name of a disease that manifests in the lips. According to the *Zhū Bìng Yuán Hòu Lùn* (vol. 30), entry on *jǐn chún* 緊唇 ("tight lips"), the Stomach Foot Yángmíng Channel begins in the nose and encircles the lips. A branch enters the spleen as a network vessel. Heat in the spleen and stomach causes qì to erupt in the lips, producing sores. If the sores are furthermore struck by the qì of wind evil or cold and dampness, this causes slight swelling and erosion, and [aversion to] cold or heat [effusion], erupting intermittently and persisting for months or even years.

4 I have added "said" because the character *yuē* 曰 is inserted here in the *Sūn Zhēn Rén* edition.

5 The intensity of classical medical treatments with moxibustion is well-known and perhaps most vividly portrayed in numerous texts and charts that outline prohibitions for burning moxa on certain locations of the body in relation to astrological events or the body's physiological changes. See for example Vivienne Lo's research on the *Huáng Dì Há Má Jīng* 《黃帝蛤蟆經》 ("Yellow Emperor's Toad Classic"), a text with illustrations that outlined prohibitions for acupuncture and moxibustion in accordance with the phases of the moon. See Vivienne Lo, "Huangdi Hama Jing (Yellow Emperor's Toad Canon)" in *Asia* Major, vol. 14, part 2, 2001..

6 See Commentary I.3

Chapter Two: Emergence Of The Newborn From The Abdomen
初生出腹第二

(2 essays on altogether 12 topics, method for predicting the newborn's longevity)

論曰:

（一）小兒初生，先以綿裹指，拭兒口中及舌上青泥惡血，此為之玉衡。

（二）若不急拭，啼聲一發，即入腹成百疾矣。

（一）兒生落地不作聲者，取暖水一器灌之，須臾當啼。

（二）兒生不作聲者，此由難產少氣故也，可取兒臍帶向身卻捋之，令氣入腹，仍呵之至百度，啼聲自發。

（三）亦可以蔥白徐徐鞭之，即啼。

Commentary II.1 ▻ Brenda Hood

落地: Within the Daoist tradition, the first cry of an infant is said to be the breaking of the microcosmic orbit (the circular cycling of qì through the Rènmài and Dūmài and marks the transition of the newborn from Earlier Heaven into the Later Heaven state. The deeper connection of the two vessels comprising the microcosmic orbit is at the uvula of the throat and the initial intake of breath and the subsequent cry open the connection and enable the infant to partake of air and food from the outside. This transition means a reorganization of function where there is now a reliance on the Lungs as a source of air qì and the Spleen/Stomach as the source of food qì rather than on being provided with all such needs through the umbilicus.

II.1 Essay

(1) When babies are just born, first take some silk floss, wrap it around a finger, and wipe away the green-blue "mud" and malign blood from the inside of the baby's mouth and the top of the tongue. This is what is called the "Jade Level."[1]

(2) If you do not wipe away [this substance] immediately, it will enter the abdomen as soon as the baby utters its first cry, and produce a hundred illnesses!

II.2 Silence Of The Newborn After Delivery

(1) If babies during delivery drop to the earth[2] without making any sound, take a bowl of warm water and pour it over them. They should cry out instantly.[3]

(2) If babies fail to make any sound after birth, this is caused by difficulties during labor and shortage of qì. You can take the baby's umbilical cord and stroke it backwards toward their body, causing qì to enter the abdomen. Now blow on them up to a hundred times,[4] and they should emit spontaneous crying sounds.

(3) You can also whip them very, very gently with the white part of a scallion, and they will cry immediately.

---

1 *Yù héng* 玉衡: An alternative edition has *xián* 銜 here instead of *héng* 衡, in which case you would translate it as "Jade Bit."

2 In the present context, *lùo dì* 落地 does not mean that the baby is accidentally dropped and therefore may have sustained injuries but rather that the baby has emerged from the womb onto this earth and that delivery is concluded. This phrase is a standard expression for the successful completion of labor, reflecting the fact that women most commonly gave birth in the squatting position. For more information on childbirth in early China, see *Qiān Jīn Fāng* vol. 2, chapters 5-8 on childbirth complications (Wilms, *Bei Ji Qian Jin Yao Fang, Volumes 2-4 on Gynecology*, pp. 180-216). See also Lee Jender, "Childbirth in Early Imperial China," (*Nan Nü* 7.2 (2005), pp. 216-286. Suffice it to say that at this point in the birth, crying is a desired manifestation of the baby's healthy respiratory functions.

3 See Commentary II.1

4 *Hē zhī* 呵之: The character used to describe this action means quite literally to exhale forcefully, perhaps even making a "he"-like sound, as you would to warm your chilled hands on a frosty morning.

（一）兒亦生，即當舉之，舉之遲晚，則令中寒，腹內雷鳴。

（二）乃先浴之，然後斷臍，不得以刀割之，須令人隔單衣物咬斷，兼以暖氣呵七遍，然後纏結，所留臍帶，令至兒足趺上。

（三）短則中寒，令兒腹中不調，常下痢。

（四）若先斷臍，然後浴者，臍中水，臍中水則發腹痛。

（五）其臍斷訖，連臍帶中多有蟲，宜急剔撥去之，不爾，入兒腹成疾。

（六）斷兒臍者，當令長六寸，長則傷肌，短則傷臟。不以時斷，若挼汁不盡，則令暖氣漸微，自生寒，令兒臍風。

II.3 Cutting The Umbilical Cord

(1) As soon as babies are born[1], immediately pick them up! If you pick them up too slowly or too late, you cause them to be struck by cold, [manifesting in] thunderous rumbling in the abdomen.

(2) Now first wash them clean and then afterwards cut the umbilical [cord]. You must not use a knife to cut it but should have a person chew it off through a single layer of cloth. At the same time, blow on it seven times with warm breath and then tie it in a knot. Have the remaining umbilical cord reach to above the baby's instep.

(3) If it is too short, it will be struck by cold, leading to disharmony inside the baby's abdomen, which manifests in constant diarrhea.

(4) If you cut the cord first and then wash the baby afterwards, you [may] get water inside the cord[2]. Water inside the cord results in episodes of abdominal pain.

(5) After the umbilical cord is severed completely, it is common to find that the [section of the] cord that connects to the navel has worms inside it. Urgently scrape them out and get rid of them, because otherwise they enter the baby's abdomen and form disease.

---

1 This reading follows the *Yī Fāng Lèi Jù* 《醫方類聚》("Categorized Collection of Medical Formulas") and most modern interpretations in reading *yì* 亦 as *yǐ* 已. This text is a medical encyclopedia in 365 volumes that was first published in 1465. While lost in China, a Japanese reprint from 1861 has preserved 266 volumes. This edition is the basis for the modern 1982 edition by *Rén mín weì shēng*. The *Sūn Zhēn Rén* edition, which contains some of the information in this section but in a very different order, has yet another version of this phrase, namely: *xiǎo ér shǐ shēng* 小兒始生... ("When babies are first born,...") instead.

2 *Qí zhōng shuǐ* 臍中水: Throughout this paragraph, *qí* 臍, which literally means "navel," is used as an abbreviation for *qí dài* 臍帶 ("umbilical cord"). You could interpret the present phrase either way.

（一）兒亦生，即當舉之，舉之遲晚，則令中寒，腹內雷鳴。

（二）乃先浴之，然後斷臍，不得以刀割之，須令人隔單衣物咬斷，兼以暖氣呵七遍，然後纏結，所留臍帶，令至兒足趺上。

（三）短則中寒，令兒腹中不調，常下痢。

（四）若先斷臍，然後浴者，臍中水，臍中水則發腹痛。

（五）其臍斷訖，連臍帶中多有蟲，宜急剔撥去之，不爾，入兒腹成疾。

（六）斷兒臍者，當令長六寸，長則傷肌，短則傷臟。不以時斷，若挼汁不盡，則令暖氣漸微，自生寒，令兒臍風。

Commentary II.2a ▻ Sabine Wilms

In classical Chinese medicine, the dreaded pediatric disease of "umbilical wind" is explained as caused by improper handling of the umbilical cord, as a result of which wind, cold, and dirty toxins invade. It manifests in symptoms like green-blue pursed lips, clenched teeth, grimacing, and in severe cases convulsions in the four extremities and arched-back rigidity. The earliest historical source of this definition is from the *Zhēn Jiǔ Jiǎ Yǐ Jīng*《針灸甲乙經》("Systematic Classic of Acupuncture and Moxibustion," composed by Huángfǔ Mì 皇甫謐 in the third century CE). The reference to umbilical wind is found in chapter 11, "Various Pediatric Diseases."

II.3 Cutting The Umbilical Cord

(6) When cutting a baby's umbilical cord, make it about 6 *cùn* in length. If it is too long, it will damage the flesh; if it is too short, it will damage the *zàng* organs. If you don't cut it in time and the fluid fails to stop flowing when you rub it, this causes the warm qì to become gradually diminished[3] and spontaneously engenders cold. This causes the baby to suffer from umbilical wind.[4]

Commentary II.2b ▻ Brenda Hood

Umbilical Wind is a disease similar to neonatal tetanus. It was recognized that the cause was improper care of the umbilicus during and after it was cut. The Míng dynasty author Wàn Quán 萬全 indicated the proper way to sever the umbilicus was to bite through it with the mouth of the biter separated from the cord with a clean cloth. The next best way was to burn it through with a hot piece of metal; and the next best way after that was to cut it with scissors and then cauterize it. After the umbilicus is cut it should then be wrapped with a soft clean cloth and allowed to dry out naturally and fall off. All Chinese texts that discuss this problem emphasize that umbilical wind is a very serious matter and should at all costs be prevented; should the problem arise, however, it must be dealt with immediately.

3 *Jiān wēi* 漸微: Alternatively, this phrase could also be interpreted as "become soaked and diminished." It is not clear to me whether the "warm qì" refers to the warm qì mentioned above, which another person is supposed to blow on the newborn baby.

4 See Commentary II.2a and Commentary II.2b

（一）生兒宜用其父故衣裹之，生女宜以其母故衣，皆勿用新帛為善。

（二）不可令衣過厚，令兒傷皮膚，害血脈，發雜瘡而黃。

（三）兒衣綿帛特忌厚熱，慎之慎之。

（四）凡小兒始生，肌膚未成，不可暖衣，暖衣則令筋骨緩弱。

II.4 Swaddling

Line II.4.1

(1) After a baby is born, use the father's old clothes to wrap them in. After a girl is born, use the mother's old clothes. In all cases, do not use new silk. This is best!

(2) Do not let the clothing be too thick because this will damage the child's skin and harm the blood and vessels, causing the outbreak of miscellaneous sores and yellowing.[1]

(3) If the baby's clothing is made with silk floss, it is particularly important to avoid thick and hot clothing. Beware! Beware!

(4) In all cases, at the beginning of a baby's life, the skin is not yet completed, and you must not dress them in warm clothes. Warm clothing causes the sinews and bones to become slack and weak.

1 *Huáng* 黄: A reference to neonatal jaundice.

（一）宜時見風日，若都不見風，則令肌膚脆軟，便易中傷。

（二）皆當以故絮衣之，勿用新綿也。

（三）凡天和暖無風之時，令母將兒於日中嬉戲，數見風日，則血凝氣剛，肌肉牢密，堪耐風寒，不致疾病。

（四）若常藏在幃帳之中，重衣溫暖，譬猶陰地之草木，不見風日，軟脆不堪風寒也。

II.4 Swaddling

Line II.4.2

(1) Expose [babies] periodically to wind and sun! If they are never exposed to wind [or sun],[1] this causes the skin to become brittle and soft, and they are then prone to damage from [cold or wind] strike.

(2) Always dress [newborn babies] in old wadding. Do not use new silk floss!

(3) Whenever the weather is mild and warm without wind, have the mother take the baby out into the sun to play. Frequent exposure to wind and sun congeals the blood, firms up the qì, and makes the flesh stout and tightly sealed. [As a result, such babies] are able to withstand wind and cold instead of falling ill.

(4) If [babies] are constantly kept behind bed curtains and warmed by double layers of clothing, they are like the grasses and trees in shady places. Not exposed to wind and sun, they are soft and brittle and [hence] unable to withstand wind and cold.

---

1 I have added "[and sun]" after the second *fēng* 風 because several of the editions and textual parallels such as the *Wài Tái Mì Yào*, as well as the following text, suggest this addition.

（一）凡裹臍法，捶治白練令柔軟，方四寸，新綿厚半寸，與帛等合之，調其緩急，急則令兒吐哯。

（二）兒生二十日，乃解視臍。

（三）若十許日兒怒啼，似衣中有刺者，此或臍燥還刺其腹，當解之，易衣更裹。

（四）裹臍時，閉戶下帳，燃火令帳中溫暖，換衣亦然，仍以溫粉粉之，此謂冬時寒也。

II.5 Wrapping The Navel

Line II.5.1

(1) For all methods of wrapping the navel, pound processed white silk until it is soft and make a square that is four *cùn* in size. Take new silk floss that is half a *cùn* thick and join [the ends] together with silk or a similar material.[1] Adjust the tightness. If it is too tight, it will make the baby vomit.

(2) No sooner than twenty days after the baby's birth, open up [the wrapping] and look at the navel.

(3) If the baby is wailing angrily after ten or more days, as if there were a thorn inside the cloth, this could mean that the cord[2] has dried up and is conversely pricking the baby's abdomen. In this case, open up the wrapping, change the dressing, and then rewrap it.

(4) When wrapping the navel, close the doors and lower the bed curtains. Burn a fire to maintain a comfortably warm temperature inside the curtains. The same applies whenever you change [the baby's] clothing. In addition, sprinkle the baby with warm powder. [These instructions] apply to cold weather in the wintertime.

---

1 In other words, stitch together both ends of the silk floss, for use as a band to wrap around the baby's abdomen and hold the cloth square in place on top of the navel.

2 While "navel" is the literal translation of *qí* 臍, in this line it obviously refers to the part of the umbilical cord that was left attached to the umbilicus after birth.

（一）若臍不愈，燒絳帛末粉之。

（二）若過一月，臍有汁不愈，燒蝦蟆灰粉之，日三四度。

（三）若臍中水及中冷，則令兒腹絞痛，夭糺啼呼，面目青黑，此是中水之過。

（四）當炙粉絮以熨之，不時治護。

II.5 Wrapping The Navel

Line II.5.2

(1) If the navel is not healing, burn crimson silk, process into a powder, and sprinkle in on.[1]

(2) If one month has passed and the navel still contains fluid and has not healed, roast a frog into ashes and use as a powder to sprinkle on the baby. [Administer this treatment] three to four times a day.

(3) If the navel is struck by water or cold, this will cause the baby to suffer from gripping pain in the abdomen, manifesting with bending over and curling up[2], wailing and crying, and a green-blue or black color in the face and eyes. This is precisely the transgression of being struck by water.

(4) Roast and pulverize [into powder] silk wadding and apply it as a hot compress. Apply this treatment at any time for protection.

---

1 The *Sūn Zhēn Rén* edition includes the following statement after this sentence: "If one month has gone by and the navel has still not healed, the nursing baby will feel greatly satiated, which causes wind in the navel."

2 Presumable a reference to neonatal intestinal colic, a common condition in infants that usually arises within the first month of life and generally disappears by the third of fourth month. It is characterized by crying, cramping, and other signs of distress in otherwise healthy infants.

（一）臍至腫者，當隨輕重。

（二）重者便灸之，乃可至八九十壯。

（三）輕者臍不大腫，但出汁，時時啼呼者，擣當歸末，和胡粉敷之。

（四）炙絮日熨之，至百日愈。以啼呼止為候。

（五）若兒糞青者，冷也，與臍中水同。

II.5 Wrapping The Navel

Line II.5.3

(1) If the navel has become swollen, proceed in accordance with the severity of the condition:

(2) In critical cases, treat it with moxibustion. You can burn up to eighty or ninety cones of moxa.

(3) In mild cases, when the navel [may] not be greatly swollen but only oozing liquid and yet the baby is crying constantly, pound *dāngguī* into a powder, mix it with *húfěn* and spread it on.

(4) Roast silk wadding and apply as a hot compress on a daily basis. After a hundred days, it will be cured. Take the fact that the baby has stopped crying as your sign [for the success of the treatment].

(5) If the baby has green-blue feces,[1] this means cold. This is identical with water inside the navel.

1 *Fèn qīng* 糞青: In the parallel phrase in the *Qiān Jīn Yì Fāng*《千金翼方》("Appended Formulas Worth a Thousand in Gold," the companion text to the *Bèi Jí Qiān Jīn Yào Fāng*, also composed by Sūn Sīmiǎo), the text has *qīng niào* 清尿 ("clear urine") instead.

甘草湯

（一）兒洗浴、斷臍竟，褓抱畢，未可與朱蜜，宜與甘草湯。

（二）以甘草如手中指一節許，打碎，以水 二合，煮取一合，以綿纏蘸取，與兒吮之。

（三）連吮汁，計得一蜆殼入腹止，兒當快吐，吐去心胸中惡汁也。

II.6 Gāncǎo Tāng (Licorice Decoction)

Line II.6.1

(1) After you have completed the washing of the [newborn] baby and the cutting of the umbilical cord, when you are done swaddling the baby, you may not yet give Zhū Mì (Cinnabar Honey).[1] It is appropriate to give Gāncǎo Tāng.

(2) Use a piece of *gāncǎo* about the length of a joint of your middle finger, crush into pieces, and boil in 2 *gě* of water until reduced to 1 *gě*. Tie up some silk floss, dip it in [the medicine], and have the baby suck on it.

(3) Have the baby continue to suck the juice and stop when you calculate that you have managed to get about a clamshell-sized amount into the abdomen. The baby should then vomit soon. The vomiting gets rid of the malign fluid in the heart and chest.

1 According to the section on neonatal care in volume 5 of the *Yī Zōng Jīn Jiàn* 《醫宗金鑒》("Golden Mirror of Orthodox Medicine"), a monumental medical compendium commissioned by the Qīng court and completed under the direction of Wú Qiānděng 吴謙等 et al. in 1742, "Zhū Mì settles the spirit and disinhibits the intestines and the stomach, is highly effective in clearing heat and preventing fright, and is also excellent for fetal heat and constipation. Be careful when using it with patients with a weak and timid constitution." Instructions for preparing Zhū Mì are found in Gé Hóng's 葛洪 *Zhǒu Hòu Bèi Jí Fāng* 《肘後備急方》("Emergency Formulas to Keep up your Sleeve," an important formula collection composed in the early fourth century BCE): "Take a piece of high-quality cinnabar, about the size of a soy bean, and grind it finely. After processing it by water grinding, make a paste by mixing it with a clamshell-sized amount of processed honey." The *Yī Zōng Jīn Jiàn* adds: "This is best taken mixed into breast milk. Do not use this if you have concerns that the baby's constitution is too weak." For the formula, see below, p. 73.

甘草湯

（一）如得吐，餘藥更不須與。若不得吐，可消息，計如飢渴，須臾更與之。

（二）若前所服及更與並不得吐者，但稍稍與之，令盡此一合止。

（三）如得吐去惡汁，令兒心神智慧無病也。

（四）飲一合盡都不吐者，是兒不含惡血耳，勿複與甘草湯，乃可與朱蜜，以鎮心神、安魂魄也。

Commentary II.3 ▻ Brenda Hood

The *hún* 魄 and *pò* 魄 are two terms in Chinese anatomy/physiology that have no equivalent in English. Classical descriptions indicate that the *hún* is housed in the Liver and the *pò* is housed in the Lung. There is a sense of pairing between the two as the *hún* is a connection to a greater consciousness acting to strategize and plan, i.e. being in the world; while the *pò* is the spirit most closely associate with the physical body, i.e. being in the body. It is thought that the *hún* can be cultivated and can leave the body (both during life and after one has died) while the *pò* is said to die with the body.

II.6 Gāncǎo Tāng (Licorice Decoction)

Line II.6.2

(1) If you were able to induce vomiting, you do not need to administer any more of the remaining medicine. If you were unable to induce vomiting, you can take a break to gauge the baby's hunger and thirst, and then in a short while give another [dose].[1]

(2) If you have still not managed to induce vomiting with the previously administered amount and the additional dose, little by little give more until you have used up this entire one *gě*, and then stop.

(3) If you were able to induce vomiting and got rid of the malign fluid, this causes the baby's heart *shén* to be full of wisdom and intelligence and to be free from illness.

(4) If a baby has drunk a full *gě* and still has not vomited at all, this means that he or she does not harbor any malign blood! Do not administer any more Gāncǎo Tāng. Now you may give Zhū Mì to settle the heart *shén* and quiet the *hún* and *pò*.[2,3]

---

1 Another dose of the same amount, or in other words, roughly equivalent to a clam-shell of liquid.

2 The *Sūn Zhēn Rén* edition adds a stern warning here: "Beware with newborn babies! You must not use counterflow moxibustion. The cruel pain [inflicted by this treatment] stirs the five vessels, and they then develop a natural tendency toward seizures. In the area between the Yellow River and the Luò River, the climate is very cold, and children have a tendency to develop tetany. On the third day after birth, people there like to administer counterflow moxibustion to prevent this. They also burn moxa on the cheeks to prevent clenched jaw.... In the area of Wú 吳 and Shǔ 蜀 (i.e., southern Jiāngsū/northern Zhèjiāng and Sìchuān, respectively), the land is damp and these conditions do not occur there. The ancient formulas are transmitted but nowadays people do not carefully differentiate between the South and the North but simply use them. Therefore, babies suffer harm."

3 See Commentary II.3

朱蜜

（一）兒新生三日中，與朱蜜者不宜多。

（二）多則冷兒，脾胃冷，腹脹，喜陰癇，氣急，變噤痙而死。

（三）新生與朱蜜法：以飛煉朱砂如大豆許，以赤蜜一蜆殼和之，以綿纏箸頭蘸取，與兒吮之。

（四）得三蘸止，一日令盡此一豆許，可三日與之，則用三豆許也。

（五）勿過此，則傷兒也。

（六）與朱蜜竟，可與牛黃如朱蜜多少也。

（七）牛黃益肝膽，除熱，定精神，止驚，辟惡氣，除小兒百病也。

II.7 Zhū Mì (Cinnabar Honey)

(1) If you do give Zhū Mì to a newborn baby within the first three days [of their life], do not give a lot.

(2) A lot [of Zhū Mì] will cool the baby down and make the spleen and stomach cool, causing abdominal distention, a tendency to yīn seizures,[1] and rapid breathing, [which can] transform into clenched jaw and tetanus, followed by death.

(3) Method for administering Zhū Mì to newborn babies: Use a roughly soybean-sized piece of cinnabar that has been refined by water grinding and mix it with a clamshell-sized amount of red honey. Wrap the tip of a chopstick with silk floss and dip it in [the honey and cinnabar mixture], soaking it up. Have the baby suck on this.

(4) Stop after you have dipped [the chopstick in the Zhū Mì] three times. In one day, use up this full amount, roughly equivalent to the size of one bean. You can give this [medicine] for three days, thus using up an amount roughly equivalent to three beans.

(5) Do not exceed this dosage, or you will harm the child.

(6) When you have finished giving the Zhū Mì, you may administer an amount of *niúhuáng* roughly equivalent to the amount of Zhū Mì.

(7) *Niúhuáng* boosts the liver and gallbladder, eliminates heat, stabilizes the *jīngshén*[2], stops fright,[3] repels malign qì, and eliminates the hundred diseases of small children.

---

1 According to the *Zhū Bìng Yuán Hòu Lùn* (vol. 45 on pediatric conditions), *xián* 癇 ("seizures") is a disease of small children that is called *diān* 癲 (translated as "withdrawal" by Wiseman) in patients older than ten *suì*. It manifests in a scrunched up face and eyes, upward-staring pupils, possibly flailing and convulsing hands and feet, rigidity in the back and spine, backward-arched neck and nape, etc. There are three types of seizures: wind seizures, which are caused by sweating due to thick clothing resulting in wind invading through the open pores; fright seizures, which are caused by great crying due to being frightened and startled; and food seizures, which are due to immoderate consumption of breast milk.

2 See Commentary II.4 on pp. 74-75 below

3 For more information on the serious neonatal condition of *jīng* 驚 ("fright") and its effects on qì, see the following chapter.

Commentary II.4 ▻ Brenda Hood

The character complex *jīngshén* 精神 has routinely in the past been translated as "spirit" as this seemed the closest English equivalent to the Chinese term. In this book, however, the complex is left as pinyin. Using the term "spirit" as a translation fails to convey the idea of two aspects acting in concert to produce an effect -- the denser more materially invested *jīng* 精 (most commonly translated as "essence") and its complement, the more rarified consciousness called *shén* 神 (most commonly translated as "spirit"). In the *Shuō Wén Jiě Zì*, *jīng* is defined as select, i.e. the cream of the crop. It is the finest of the fine and has come to refer to the very essence of something. It includes within its component parts the radical for rice and the component for green, the color associated with Wood, the generating aspect of the five phases cycle. Extended meanings of the character in the context of Chinese medicine include the concept of semen and the sense that it forms a basis for the production or generation of something. In the *Shuō Wén Jiě Zì*, *shén* 神 is defined as 天神，引出萬物者也: "Heavenly *shén*-spirit draws out the 10,000 things." I interpret this as meaning that a higher order of consciousness draws out or makes manifest the phenomena that make up the world. The character *shén* 神 itself is a combination of two components. The first is *shì* 示 and in the *Shuō Wén* means: 天垂象，見吉凶，所以示人也。从二。三垂，日月星也。觀乎天文，以察時變。示，神事也。"Images suspended from Heaven, [enabling] observation of auspicious and inauspicious to show humankind... The three suspensions are the sun, the moon, and the stars. Observation of Heaven's writings enables one to investigate the changes of the seasons. *Shì* 示 refers to spiritual affairs." In other words, something is made manifest so that one might see its goodness or badness, implying a consciousness and an ability to be attracted or repulsed by what is perceived. The second component is *shēn* 申. In the *Shuō Wén* it is defined as: 神也。七月，陰气成，體自申束。从臼，自持也。吏臣餔時聽事，申旦政也。"*Shén*-spirit. In the seventh month, yīn qì completes (begins to rise) and the body is gathered in by *shēn* (the seventh Earthly branch). [This character] is formed from the components for mortar and self-holding. When the ambassadors and counselors meet to eat, they listen to affairs [of the country] and [thus] *shēn* refers to the morning administration." From this definition one can see the elements of holding within a container and the administration of the material. Together with the first component of the character, the meaning of *shén* 神 becomes so much more than can be conveyed by the English word "spirit." We have also decided to not translate the term as "essence spirit," as is now becoming more common in more recent translations, because this too is insufficient to convey the meanings of the character complex let alone its subtle nuances.

If one were to give a simple definition of the character complex *jīngshén*, it could be said that it is the end result of the interaction of the essence of form and the administration of the spirit over that container. It is, as all things in Chinese medicine turn out to be, a complex formed by the interaction of yīn and yáng and the manifestation of that interaction, perceivable by the observer practitioner, is how we know the relative health of the individual.

Throughout the text, it will be useful for the reader to consider what the qì mechanism/dynamic is doing or how it is being affected by the practices described. It will also help to know that the underlying logic of the processes.

（一）新生三日後，應開腸胃，助穀神。

（二）可研米作厚飲，如乳酪厚薄，以豆大與兒咽之，頻咽三豆許止，日三與之，滿七日可與哺也。

（三）兒生十日始哺如棗核，二十日倍之，五十日如彈丸，百日如棗。

（四）若乳汁少，不得从此法，當用意小增之。

II.8 Feeding Babies

Line II.8.1

(1) After the third day after birth, you should open up the [newborn child's] intestines and stomach to assist the grain *shén*.

(2) You can grind [uncooked] rice to make a thick drink with a consistency like curdled milk, and give [babies] bean-sized amounts to swallow. Repeatedly make them swallow an amount equivalent to about three beans, and then stop. Give this [rice drink] three times a day. You can feed this for a full seven days.[1]

(3) On the tenth day after birth, begin feeding amounts about the size of a jujube pit.[2] Twenty days after birth, double [the amount]. Fifty days after birth, feed pellet-sized amounts, and a hundred days after birth, feed jujube-sized amounts.

(4) If the breast milk is scanty,[3] you cannot follow this method, but should use your best judgment to increase it slightly.

---

1 Or should this be interpreted as a separate sentence, as "After a full seven days, you may feed [the baby]"? The interpretation of this line depends to a large extent on whether you read the following instructions as still referring to feeding rice milk in subtly increasing amounts or whether you interpret them as separate statements, referring to feeding infants anything besides breast milk. If you read them as separate lines, you are confronted with an apparent contradiction, since the first line instructs the reader to start feeding rice milk after 3 days but the following line specifies the tenth day as the time to begin supplemental feeding. One possible explanation would be that the first phrase refers simply to rice drink as a treatment for opening up the intestines and stomach, while the third phrase refers to actually feeding the baby solid food in general, or in other words anything besides breast milk as nourishment, as opposed to the small amounts of medicinal preparations like the rice drink or the Zhū Mì mentioned in the preceding section.

2 In the standard modern editions, based on the Sòng revisions by Lín Yī and his team, this line is interpreted as being a part of the previous section on the supplemental feeding of ground rice milk. In the *Sūn Zhēn Rén* edition, however, this line is a separate paragraph, unrelated to the section on rice milk. As such, it does not relate specifically to feeding rice milk but refers to feeding newborn babies anything besides breast milk. In either reading, this set of instructions appears to contradict the following line, which warns against the dangers of introducing supplemental food too early.

3 The *Sūn Zhēn Rén* edition adds here "and does not flow through" (*bù tōng* 不通), or in other words, if the mother is suffering from agalactia.

（一）若三十日而哺者，令兒無疾。

（二）兒哺早者，兒不勝穀氣，令生病，頭面身體喜生瘡，愈而複發，令兒尪弱難養。

（三）三十日後雖哺勿多，若不嗜食，勿強與之。

（四）強與之不消，複生疾病。

（五）哺乳不進者，腹中皆有痰癖也。

（六）當以四物紫丸微下之，節哺乳，數日便自愈。

（七）小兒微寒熱，亦當爾利之，要當下之，然後乃瘥。

II.8 Feeding Babies

Line II.8.2

(1) If you [wait] for thirty days [after birth] and only then feed [anything besides breast milk], this will cause the child to be free from disease.[1]

(2) If you introduce food to babies too early, they cannot overcome the qì of grain, which will cause the formation of diseases. On the head, face, and body, they will have a tendency to engender sores that will heal and then erupt again. This makes babies small and weak and difficult to nourish.

(3) After thirty days, even though you may now give them food [other than breast milk], do not feed them a lot. If they do not have a strong desire for food, do not force it on them.

(4) If you force-feed them and they fail to disperse [the food],[2] you again engender disease.

(5) If [supplemental] food and breast milk fail to enter [into the baby's body], it always means the presence of phlegm aggregations in the abdomen.[3]

(6) Use Sì Wù Zǐ Wán (Four Substances Purple Pill) to induce a mild downward action. Regulate nursing and feeding, and after a number of days the baby will recover naturally.

(7) If babies suffer from slight cold or heat, you must also disinhibit [the heat or cold] like this. It is essential that you induce a downward movement [to eliminate it], because recovery will occur only after this.

---

1 My reading here is based on a sentence preceding this phrase in the *Sūn Zhēn Rén* edition, which states: "Small children must live out a full thirty days before you may feed them [supplemental food]."

2 Dispersal of food here means that they are unable to digest the food, with the result that it stagnates in the abdomen.

3 The *Sūn Zhēn Rén* edition has instead: "If babies are unable to nurse or eat, Zǐ Shuāng Wán 紫雙丸 (Purple Double Pill) should be used to induce a downward action. [In this type of] small children, the qì is overabundant and they have a disease, so you must bring it down, but you may not injure them."

（一）凡乳兒不欲太飽，飽則嘔吐。

（二）每候兒吐者，乳太飽也，以空乳乳之即消，日四。

（三）乳兒若臍未愈，乳兒太飽，令風中臍也。

（四）夏不去熱乳，令兒嘔逆。冬不去寒乳，令兒咳痢。

II.9 Overeating And Other Breastfeeding Problems

Line II.9.1

(1) Whenever you are breastfeeding a baby, you never want them to eat until they are too full. Overeating results in retching and vomiting.

(2) Every time you encounter the symptom of vomiting in babies, it means that they are over-satiated on breast milk. Nurse them on an empty breast, to make the [already ingested] milk disperse.[1] Do this four times a day.

(3) In breastfeeding babies, if their navel has not healed yet and you let them nurse until they are overly full, this allows wind to strike the navel.

(4) In the summertime, if you do not get rid of the heat in the breast,[2] this causes babies to suffer from retching and counterflow. In the wintertime, if you do not get rid of the cold in the breast, this causes babies to suffer from cough and dysentery.[3]

---

1 This means that they will digest what they have ingested, which will prevent the formation of pathological accumulations and aggregations over time.

2 "Getting rid of the heat in the breast" presumably means to dispose of milk that is too hot in temperature. In an alternative interpretation, we could read this passage as "If you do not get rid of hot breasts,..." which could possibly refer to cooling (or in the case of winter, warming) the breast before allowing the baby to nurse. It seems more likely to me, however, that this line instructs the mother or wet nurse to squirt out the first bit of milk that is right by the nipple and therefore colder or hotter in temperature than the rest of the milk that is deeper inside the breast and therefore insulated from the extremes of the outside temperature.

3 The *Sūn Zhēn Rén* edition has "diarrhea" (*lì* 利) instead. The two characters *lì* 利 and *lì* 痢 are often used interchangeably in the various editions. See Commentary III.9 on p. 132 for further explanation.

（一）母新房以乳兒，令兒羸瘦，交脛不能行。

（二）母有熱以乳兒，令變黃、不能食。

（三）母怒以乳兒，令喜驚、發氣疝，又令上氣癲狂。

（四）母新吐下以乳兒，令虛羸。

（五）母醉以乳兒，令身熱腹滿。

Commentary II.5 ▻ Sabine Wilms

Shàn 疝 is a common technical term in Chinese medicine, translated by Wiseman as "mounting" but in modern TCM generally equated with the biomedical condition of hernia. Wiseman makes a convincing case that it is historically incorrect to equate *shàn* directly with "hernia" in all cases, since the conditions overlap but *shàn* can also refer to numerous other pathologies that do not involve the biomedical condition of hernia. *Qì shàn* 氣疝 ("Qì-type *shàn*) is a form of *shàn* that is explained in the *Zhū Bìng Yuán Hòu Lùn* (vol. 20, entry on "Seven Types of *Shàn*") as being characterized by abruptly alternating fullness and decrease, leading to pain. The entry on "The Various Types of *Shàn*" in the same volume describes all forms of *shàn* as "caused by yīn qì gathering inside, compounded by cold qì. As a result, *yíng* provisioning and *wèi* defense are out of balance, blood and qì are weak, and wind and cold are able to enter the abdomen to engender *shàn*. *Shàn* means pain. It can be pain in the lesser abdomen, with inability to defecate or urinate. Or it can be reversal cold in the hands and feet and around the navel, with discharge of white sweat. Or it can be cold qì rising counterflow to prod the heart and abdomen, causing heart pain. Or it can be abdominal urgency with abdominal pain. All of these are different but all are called *shàn*. They are characterized by a string-like tight pulse." With slight hesitation, I have chosen to translate *shàn* above as "hernia" because that is clearly what it refers to in the current context. In the line above, "abruptly alternative fullness and decrease" refers to the intestines bulging out and returning back. Hernias are a common condition particularly in male infants.

II.9 Overeating And Other Breastfeeding Problems

Line II.9.2

(1) If a mother nurses a baby in a new building, the baby will suffer from marked emaciation and crossed shinbones, resulting in failure to walk.

(2) If a mother has heat [in her body] and nurses a baby in this condition, this causes [the baby] to turn yellow and be unable to eat.

(3) If a mother is angry and nurses a baby in this condition, the results [in the baby] are a tendency to fright and the eruption of hernias[1] while also causing qì ascent and *diān* insanity and *kuáng* mania.

(4) If a mother has recently suffered from vomiting or diarrhea and nurses a baby in this condition, this causes vacuity and emaciation [in the baby].

(5) If a mother is inebriated and nurses a baby in this condition, this causes generalized heat and abdominal fullness [in the baby].

---

1 See Commentary II.5

凡新生小兒，一月內常飲豬乳大佳。

（一）凡乳母乳兒，當先極挼，散其熱氣，勿令汁奔出，令兒噎，輒奪其乳，令得息，息已，複乳之。

（二）如是十返五返，視兒飢飽節度，知一日中幾乳而足，以為常。

（三）又常捉去宿乳。

（四）兒若臥，乳母當以臂枕之，令乳與兒頭平乃乳之，令兒不噎。

（五）母欲寐，則奪其乳，恐填口鼻，又不知飢飽也。

II.10 Feeding Sow's Milk

For all newborn babies, it is of great benefit to frequently drink sow's milk in the first month [after birth].

II.11 Proper Breastfeeding

(1) Whenever wet nurses breastfeed a baby, they must first rub [their breasts] thoroughly to dissipate their hot qì. Do not allow the milk to pour out in a torrent because this causes the baby to hiccup. Quickly snatch the breast away [from the baby] and make [the milk] stop [flowing]. Once it has stopped, start nursing again.

(2) Proceed like this over and over numerous times and see to it that the baby is neither over-satiated nor starved but is nursing in moderation. Be conscious of how many times the baby has nursed in one day and have it be enough. Make this consistent.

(3) Moreover, consistently capture and dispose of the overnight breast milk.[1]

(4) With the baby lying in a cradled position, the wet nurse should use her arm as a pillow [for the baby's head] in such a way that the breast and the baby's head are level, and only then nurse the baby. This causes the baby to not suffer from hiccup.

(5) When the mother[2] is about to fall asleep, [she must] take the breast away, for fear that [the milk] could plug up the baby's mouth or nose. Moreover, you will not know whether the baby has eaten too much or too little.

---

1 This is a reference to the milk that has accumulated in the wet nurse's breasts overnight.

2 This term could refer here either literally to the birth mother, but more likely, given the context of this whole paragraph, to the wet nurse, in Chinese referred to as "nursing mother" (*rǔ mǔ* 乳母).

浴兒法

（一）凡浴小兒，湯極須令冷熱調和。冷熱失所，令兒驚，亦致五臟之疾也。

（二）凡兒冬不可久浴，浴久則傷寒。夏不可久浴，浴久則傷熱。

（三）數浴背冷，則發癇。若不浴，又令兒毛落。

（四）新生浴兒者，以豬膽一枚，取汁投湯中以浴兒，終身不患瘡疥。

（五）勿以雜水浴之。

II.12 How To Bathe Babies

(1) Whenever you bathe a baby, it is always of utmost importance that the temperature of the bathwater be adjusted so that it is just right. If it is either too hot or too cold, this causes fright in the baby, as well as leading to disease in the five *zàng* organs.

(2) In the winter, you must never bathe babies for a long time. If you bathe them for a long time, they will suffer cold damage. In the summer, you may not bathe them for a long time either.[1] If you bathe them for a long time, they will suffer heat damage.

(3) If you bathe them too frequently and the back gets cold, seizures result. If you do not bathe them, on the other hand, you cause the body hair to fall out.

(4) Whenever you bathe newborn babies, take one pig's gallbladder, remove the liquid, and add that to the bathwater. If you bathe babies in this, they will not suffer from sores and scabs for the rest of their life.

(5) Do not bathe babies in impure water.[2]

1 In an interesting twist on this line, the *Sūn Zhēn Rén* edition has instead: *xià bù kě bù yù* 夏不可不浴 ("In the summer you may not forego washing them"). It is interesting that none of the modern editions mentions this major discrepancy.
2 The character *zá* 雜 literally describes the state of having all five colors mixed together (*Shuō Wén*: *wǔ cǎi xiāng hé yě* 五采相合也), but here simply means water that has been contaminated. One possible narrower meaning of the character is as a synonym for *cè* 廁 ("latrine"), in which case the compound *zá shuǐ* 雜水 would mean "latrine water," or water contaminated by human waste.

桃根湯

（一）兒生三日，宜用桃根湯浴。

（二）桃根、李根、梅根各二兩，枝亦得。

（三）㕮咀之，以水三斗，煮二十沸，去滓。

（四）浴兒良，去不祥，令兒終身無瘡疥。

金虎湯

（一）治小兒驚，辟惡氣，以金虎湯浴。

（二）金一斤，虎頭骨一枚，以水三斗，煮為湯浴。

（三）但須浴即煮用之。

II.13 Táogēn Tāng (Peach Root Decoction)

(1) On the third day after the baby's birth, it is appropriate to use Táogēn Tāng to bathe them.

(2) Use two *liǎng* each of *táogēn, lǐgēn,* and *méigēn.*[1] You may also use the branches.

(3) Pound[2] them and decoct in three *dǒu* of water, bringing the mixture to a boil twenty times. Remove the dregs.

(4) Bathing babies [in this decoction] is excellent. It gets rid of inauspicious things and allows them to not suffer from sores and scales for the rest of their life.

II.14 Jīn Hǔ Tāng (Gold Tiger Decoction)

(1) To treat fright in small children and to avoid malign qì, bathe them in Jīn Hǔ Tāng.

(2) Take one *jīn* of gold and one tiger skull and decoct these in three *dǒu* of water to make a bathing decoction.

(3) But you must wait until you [are ready for] the bath and then decoct it for immediate use.[3]

---

1 See the Single Herb and Formula index on page 295 for more detail.

2 *Fǔ jǔ* 㕮咀: This compound is a common technical term referring to a specific method of preparing medicinals. Literally meaning "to chew," Donald Harper still translates it as such for the early Hàn period in his translation of the Mǎwāngduī medical manuscripts, but Sūn Sīmiǎo specifically states in the instructions on compounding medicines in the first volume of the *Qiān Jīn Fāng*: "Whenever [compounding] medicinal decoctions, wines, or pastes, when the ancient prescriptions all state to chew [the ingredients], it means to pound them all to the size of soybeans and blow on them to remove the fine powder."

3 It is very interesting that the parallel prescription in the *Sūn Zhēn Rén* edition is almost literally identical but uses not a tiger's skull but "skulls from large insects" (*dà chóng tóu gǔ* 大蟲頭骨) instead.

（一）凡小兒初出腹有鵝口者，其舌上有白屑如米，劇者鼻外亦有之。

（二）此由兒在胞胎中受穀氣盛故也，或妊娠時嗜糯米使之然。

（三）治之法：以髮纏箸頭，蘸井花水撩拭之，三日如此，便脫去也。

（四）如不脫，可煮栗荴汁令濃，以綿纏箸頭拭之。

（五）若春夏無栗荴，可煮栗木皮，如用井花水法。

Commentary II.6 ▻ Sabine Wilms

The *Zhū Bìng Yuán Hòu Lùn*, vol. 50 explains this condition as follows: "Whenever newborn babies have little white pieces in their mouth that spread to the top of the tongue forming sores there that resemble the inside of a goose's mouth, it is referred to as 'goose mouth.' This condition is due to the fact that the child received an overabundance of grain qì during the fetal stage, causing heat qì in the heart and spleen. Steaming upward, this heat qì breaks out in the mouth." The condition is also known as *xuě kǒu* 雪口 ("snow mouth").

Commentary II.7 ▻ Sabine Wilms

井花水 *jǐng huā shuǐ*: This is the first water drawn from a well at dawn. In the *Běn Cǎo Gāng Mù* (vol. 5, entry 15), it is listed as a synonym under *jǐng quán shuǐ* 井泉水 ("well spring water"). A common ingredient in Daoist alchemy, this type of well water has many medicinal applications. The best grade comes from deep wells that tap into the veins in the earth, rather than drawing their water from nearby rivers or lakes. According to Yú Tuán 虞摶, a physician active in the early sixteenth century, it is ideal for decocting medicinals that replenish yīn and for refining alchemical preparations since it contains the first true qì of Heaven that floats on the water's surface (quoted in *Běn Cǎo Gāng Mù* 5:15).

II.15 Treatment For Thrush

(1) If babies suffer from thrush[1] when they first emerge from the [mother's] abdomen, they invariably have little white pieces like rice grains on their tongue. In severe cases, these are also present on the outside of the nose.[2]

(2) This condition is caused by the fact that the baby received an overabundance of grain qì while in utero. Alternatively, it can also come about because [the mother] was addicted to glutinous rice during pregnancy.

(3) Treatment method: Take human hair and wrap around the tip of a chopstick. Dip in well-flower water[3] and sprinkle and wipe [the water] on [the affected areas]. Proceed like this for three days, and you will get rid of it.

(4) If you fail to get rid of it [by this method], you can decoct chestnut skins[4] until the liquid thickens. Wrap the tip of a chopstick with silk floss and use this to wipe it on [the affected area].

(5) If it is spring or summer and you don't have chestnut skins, you can decoct the bark from chestnut trees [and proceed] in the manner described above for using well-flower water.

---

1 See Commentary II.6

2 An alternate version of the text instead says, "These are also present inside the nose."

3 See Commentary II.7

4 Strictly speaking, *lì fú* 栗荴 refers to the membrane between the nut and the shell in chestnuts. Wiseman therefore translates it as "chestnut endocarp."

（一）小兒初出腹有連舌，舌下有膜如石榴子中隔，連其舌下後，喜令兒言語不發不轉也。

（二）可以爪摘斷之，微有血出，無害。

（三）若血出不止，可燒髮作灰末，敷之，血便止也。

II.16 Treatment For Connected Tongue

(1) If babies suffer from "connected tongue"[1] when they first emerge from the [mother's] abdomen, there is a membrane underneath the tongue that resembles the dividing walls between seeds inside a pomegranate. When a baby's tongue is tied down [like this], there is a tendency for the baby to be unable to emit sounds or transmit speech.

(2) You can use a pincer to pick up the tongue and sever [the membrane]. There will be slight bleeding, but this is not harmful.

(3) If the bleeding does not stop, you can roast head hair into ashes and pulverize it. Spread this on [the bleeding wound], and the bleeding will then stop.

1 This refers to a neonatal condition where the tongue is connected to the floor of the mouth because the length of the frenulum is insufficient. The biomedical term for this condition is ankyloglossia.

（一）小兒出腹六七日後，其血氣收斂成肉，則口、舌、喉、頰裡清淨也。

（二）若喉裡舌上有物，如蘆籜盛水狀者，若懸癰有脹起者，可以綿纏長針，留刃處如粟米許大。

（三）以刺決之，令氣泄，去青黃赤血汁也。

（四）一刺之止，消息一日，未消者，來日又刺之，不過三刺自消盡。

（五）餘小小未消，三刺亦止，自然得消也。

（一）有著舌下如此者，名重舌。

（二）有著頰裡及上腭如此者，名重腭。

（三）有著齒齦上者，名重齦。

（四）皆刺去血汁也。

II.17 Treatment For Hanging Welling-Abscesses

Line II.17.1

(1) On the sixth or seventh day after babies have emerged from the [mother's] abdomen, their blood and qì contract and form flesh. As a result, the insides of the mouth, tongue, throat, and cheeks become clean.

(2) If there is something inside the throat or on top of the tongue that looks like a sheath of reed that is holding water,[1] or if there is a hanging welling-abscess with swelling and protrusion, you can wrap a large needle with silk floss, leaving a space open for the blade about the size of a millet grain.

(3) Use this [tool] to prick [the abscess] and break it open, allowing the qì to drain. Get rid of the green-blue, yellow, or red blood and fluids.

(4) Prick it once and stop. Let it rest for one day. If it is not dispersed yet, prick it again on the following day. With no more than three prickings, it will completely disperse on its own.

(5) If there is a tiny bit left over that fails to disperse, still stop after three prickings. Leave it alone, and it will disperse on its own.

Line II.17.2

(1) If there is something attached to the underside of the tongue like this, it is called "double tongue."

(2) If there is something attached to the inside of the cheek and on top of the palate like this, it is called "double palate."

(3) If there is something attached to the top of the gums, it is called "double gums."

(4) In all cases, prick it to get rid of the blood and fluids.

---

1 The *Sūn Zhēn Rén* edition is quite a bit different here, having *chéng* 成 instead of *shèng* 盛: "If there is something inside the throat or on top of the tongue that looks like a sheath of reed and is producing water, it is called hanging welling-abscess. The presence of qì is causing swelling and protrusion." On the other hand, the character 成 is often used as an alternate character for 盛.

小兒生輒死治之法

(一) 當候視兒口中懸癰前上腭有泡者，以指摘取頭，決令潰去血。

(二) 勿令血入咽，入咽殺兒，急急慎之。

(三) 小兒初出腹，骨肉未斂，肌肉猶是血也，血凝乃堅成肌肉耳。

(四) 其血沮敗不成肌肉，則使面目繞鼻口左右悉黄而啼，閉目，聚口，撮面，口中乾燥，四肢不能伸縮者，皆是血脈不斂也，喜不育。

(五) 若有如此者，皆宜與龍膽湯也。

Commentary II.8 ▻Brenda Hood

When considering the words of Sūn Sīmiǎo, it is necessary to think about what the qì dynamic is doing in the newborn. All aspects of a newborn are in the phase of growth. On the surface this seems to be an expansive action and in fact the end result is physical growth and mature functioning. However, in order to achieve growth, there must be a drawing in and consolidating first. One cannot build a house without first bringing in the materials required and then arranging them. In this respect, the drawing-in actions of the organs and, in this instance bones, are primary in the newborn, and disruption to this action as seen in fright seizures (described in the next chapter) is like accumulating materials to build a house and then having a tornado run through the site throwing around all the materials intended for use the next day in the building. In this example, the building materials are lost and/or damaged, with the end result that the building cannot proceed as planned or perhaps even at all.

II.18 How To Treat Sudden Neonatal Death

(1) Check for signs by seeing whether there are blisters on the palate in front of or above a hanging welling-abscess inside the baby's mouth. Use your finger to "pluck" them and dispose of the head. Break them open so that they burst and get rid of the blood.

(2) Do not allow the blood to run into the throat. If it runs into the throat, it will kill the baby. Quickly, quickly! Beware of this!

(3) When babies first emerge from the [mother's] abdomen, the bones and flesh are not yet drawn in[1]. The flesh is still just blood. As the blood congeals, it becomes firm and forms flesh.

(4) If this blood spoils instead of forming flesh, it causes thorough yellowing in the face and eyes, encircling the nose, and to both sides of the mouth, accompanied by wailing, closed eyes, a puckered mouth and pinched face, dryness in the mouth, and inability to extend or contract the four limbs. All [these symptoms] mean that the blood in the vessels has failed to be drawn in and that there is a tendency to die prematurely.

(5) If a baby shows symptoms like these, always administer Lóngdǎn Tāng.[2]

---

1 See Commentary II.8

2 The formula for Lóngdǎn Tāng 龍膽湯 (Gentian Decoction) is found further down in the present volume in chapter 3 "Fright Seizures" on pages 151-153.

相兒命短長法

（一）兒初生，叫聲連延相屬者，壽。

（二）聲絕而複揚急者，不壽。

（三）啼聲散，不成人。

（四）啼聲深，不成人。

（五）臍中無血者，好。

（六）臍小者，不壽。

（七）通身軟弱如無骨者，不壽。

（八）鮮白長大者，壽。

II.19 How To Foretell The Length Of A Baby's Life

Line II.19.1

(1) When babies are first born, if they cry out with a long continuous wail, this means longevity.

(2) If the cry is interrupted but then rises again with urgency, this means no longevity.

(3) If the sound of the cry is scattered, such babies will not live to adulthood.[1]

(4) If the sound of the cry is deep, such babies will not live to adulthood.

(5) If there is no blood in the navel,[2] this is good.

(6) If the navel is small, this means no longevity.

(7) If babies are soft and weak in the entire body, as if without bones, this means no longevity.

(8) If babies are fresh white [in complexion] and grown large, this means longevity.

---

1 *Bù chéng rén* 不成人: While this expression can also refer to a person who fails to become successful later in life or to a vile, low-quality person of loose morals, I choose to read it more literally here and in its original meaning, that the child will not complete his or her development to complete adulthood. As another alternative, it could mean to suffer from physical defects, in the sense of becoming a less than perfect person, a person with defects.

2 This could also refer to the umbilical cord (literally: *qí dài* 臍帶), which is also abbreviated in several instances above simply as *qí* 臍.

相兒命短長法

（一）自開目者，不成人。

（二）目視不正，數動者，大非佳。

（三）汗血者，多厄不壽。

（四）汗不流，不成人。

（五）小便凝如脂膏，不成人。

（六）頭四破，不成人。

（七）常搖手足者，不成人。

（八）早坐、早行、早齒、早語，皆惡性，非佳人。

II.19 How To Foretell The Length Of A Baby's Life

Line II.19.2

(1) If they open their eyes spontaneously, they will not live to adulthood.

(2) If the eyes do not look straight ahead but move frequently, they will surely not become a good [person].[1]

(3) If they sweat blood, this means many disasters and no longevity.

(4) If the sweat fails to flow, they will not live to adulthood.

(5) If the urine is congealed like lard or paste, they will not live to adulthood.

(6) If the head is broken on all four sides, they will not live to adulthood.

(7) If they constantly shake their hands and feet, they will not live to adulthood.

(8) Sitting up early, walking early, teething early, and speaking early, these all [indicate] a malicious nature. Such babies will not become good persons.

1 My interpretation of *jiā* 佳 as "goodness" in the moral sense of the word is based on the *Shuō Wén* definition as *shàn* 善, and on its contrast in the following section with *è xìng* 惡性 (malicious nature).

相兒命短長法

（一）頭毛不周匝者，不成人。

（二）髮稀少者，強不聽人。

（三）額上有旋毛，早貴，妨父母。

（四）兒生枕骨不成者，能言而死。

（五）尻骨不成者，能倨而死。

（六）掌骨不成者，能匍匐而死。

（七）踵骨不成者，能行而死。

（八）臏骨不成者，能立而死。

II.19 How To Foretell The Length Of A Baby's Life

Line II.19.3

(1) If the hair on the head does not cover the head all around, such babies will not live to adulthood.

(2) If the hair on the head is scant, they will be forceful and not listen to others.

(3) The presence of twirling hairs on top of the forehead means early riches but a hindrance to the parents.

(4) If babies are born with an incompletely formed occipital bone, they will die by the time they are able to speak.

(5) If the coccyx is not completely formed, they will die by the time they are able to sit up.

(6) If the bones in the palm of the hand are not completely formed, they will die by the time they are able to crawl.

(7) If the heels are not completely formed, they will die by the time they are able to walk.

(8) If the knees are not completely formed, they will die by the time they are able to stand up.

相兒命短長法

（一）身不收者，死。

（二）魚口者，死。

（三）股間無生肉者，死。

（四）頤下破者，死。

（五）陰不起者，死。

（六）陰囊下白者，死；赤者，死。

（七）卵縫通達，黑者，壽。

II.19 How To Foretell The Length Of A Baby's Life

Line II.19.4

(1) Inability to contract the body means death.

(2) A fish mouth[1] means death.

(3) Failure to engender flesh in the thighs means death.

(4) Brokenness below the cheeks[2] means death.

(5) If the penis fails to rise, this means death.

(6) Whiteness below the scrotum means death. Redness means death.

(7) When the seam in the middle of the scrotum reaches all the way and is black, this means longevity.

---

1 *Yú kǒu* 魚口: This refers to a localized ulceration in the groin, when the lymph nodes there start suppurating. The name is said to be derived from the uneven shape of the wound, which is open or closed depending on the person's anatomical features. Alternatively, it could possibly refer literally to a mouth in the shape of a fish's mouth.

2 According to Lillian Pearl Bridges, expert in the ancient Chinese science of face reading and author of *Face Reading in Chinese Medicine* (Churchill Livingstone, 2003, 2nd edition by Elsevier, 2012), this means that the Breath of Life area, the place that becomes hollow when you suck in your cheeks, is sunken and usually dark. It is an indication of severe lung deficiency and therefore means imminent death in newborns! The "brokenness" here refers to the break in the plane of the skin, which is supposed to be plump and full.

論曰:

（一）兒三歲以上，十歲以下，視其性氣高下，即可知其夭壽大略。

（二）兒小時識悟通敏過人者多夭，大則項託、顏回之流是也。

（三）小兒骨法：成就威儀，回轉遲舒，稍費人精神雕琢者壽。

（四）其預知人意，回旋敏速者，亦夭，即楊修、孔融之徒是也。

（一）由此觀之，夭壽大略可知也。

（二）亦猶梅花早發，不睹歲寒。甘菊晚成,終於年事。是知晚成者，壽之兆也。

II.20 Essay

Line II.20.1

(1) In children between the ages of three and ten *suì*, you can get a general idea about the length of their life by observing whether their character and qì are elevated or inferior.

(2) Children who have a high level of knowledge and insight and are intelligent beyond their peers are more likely to die prematurely. The reason for this is that when they grow up, they will follow the path of Xiàng Tuō and Yán Huí.[1]

(3) Method of [divining] small children by the bones: If they respond to success in a dignified manner, are slow when turning around to look back, expend little on other people, and have an *jīngshén* like polished jade, this means longevity.

(4) When they know other people's intentions in advance and maneuver with speed and agility, this also means a short life. The reason for this is that they will follow the footsteps of Yáng Xiū and Kǒng Róng.[2]

Line II.20.2

(1) If you observe [babies] on the basis of these [guidelines], you can get a general idea about their short or long life.

(2) This is just like the early blossoming of the plum flowers, without regard for the harshness of winter. [By contrast,] the sweet chrysanthemum matures late, at the very end of its life. This is how you know that maturing late is a predictor of longevity.

---

1 These are two famous child prodigies who died at a very young age.

2 These are two famous intellectuals who were born during the Hàn dynasty but were killed by Cáo Cāo 曹操 after angering him.

Chapter Three: Fright Seizures
驚癇第三

(3 essays, 1 method of diagnosing seizures, 13 formulas, 23 moxibustion methods)

論曰:

(一) 少小所以有癇病及痓病者，皆由臟氣不平故也。

(二) 新生即癇者，是其五臟不收斂，血氣不聚，五脈不流，骨怯不成也，多不全育。

(三) 其一月四十日以上至期歲而癇者，亦由乳養失理，血氣不和，風邪所中也。

(四) 病先身熱掣瘲、驚啼叫喚，而後發癇，脈浮者為陽癇。病在六腑，外在肌膚，猶易治也

(五) 病先身冷、不驚掣、不啼呼、而病發時脈沉者，為陰癇。病在五臟，內在骨髓，極難治也。

Commentary III.1 ▻ Brenda Hood

Sù Wèn (素問) 3 states : 故陽強不能密，陰氣乃絕，陰平陽秘，精神乃治，陰陽離決，精氣乃絕. My translation of this quote is: "[If] yáng is powerful it cannot be dense (coherent) and yīn will thus end; [if] yīn is smooth and yáng is dense, then *jīngshén* can thereof be treated. [If] yīn and yáng separate, then *jīngshén* will thereof end." This quote reflects the idea that there needs to be organization and coherence between the two polar aspects that make up an organism and that there needs be a balance with neither of them too strong or in excess nor too weak or deficient. According to the quote, yīn needs to be internally coherent or smooth -- kind of like a sandbox where the sand is all shaken smooth and each grain of sand is in coherent organization with all of the other grains of sand. Yáng, on the other hand, needs to have a certain density or power but one that is not overpowering, in order to make things function properly. The passage in the *Qiān Jīn Fāng* states: "臟气不平", translated as "visceral qì is not even." This is a variation of the quote from *Sù Wèn* 3 and refers to the idea that in children, who are considered more purely yáng in nature, yáng qì and in this case specifically visceral qì which is yáng in nature, can operate in an unsmooth way, perhaps referring to operating in fits and starts rather than a smooth flow. It is precisely this kind of a pathology that can manifest in seizures and tetany.

III.1 Essay

Line III.1.1 Causes and Forms of Seizures

(1) The reason why seizures and tetany occur in very early childhood is always that visceral qì is not even.[1]

(2) When seizures occur immediately after birth, this means that the baby's five *zàng* organs are failing to contract, the blood and qì are failing to gather, there is no flow in the five vessels, and the bones are timid and incomplete.[2] In the majority of cases, [such babies] will not develop completely.[3]

(3) When the seizures occur between the first month or 40 days and the end of the first full year of life, they can also be caused by disorderly breastfeeding or nurturing, disharmony of blood and qì, or by being struck by wind evil.[4]

(4) In cases where this disease manifests first with generalized heat, tugging and slackening, and frightful wailing and crying, and only afterwards with episodes of seizures, [during which the patient has] a floating pulse, this means yáng seizures. [In such cases,] the disease is located in the six *fǔ* organs and on the outside in the skin, and is still easy to treat.

(5) In cases where this disease manifests first with generalized cold, no frightful tugging, no wailing and crying, and then, when the disease breaks out, with a sunken pulse, this means yīn seizures. [In such cases,] the disease is located in the five *zàng* organs and on the inside in the bones and marrow, and is extremely difficult to treat.

---

1 See Commentary III.1

2 See Commentary III.2

3 *Quán yù* 全育: In medieval China, a child's inability to mature fully meant most likely that he or she was unable to live to adulthood.

4 The *Sūn Zhēn Rén* edition has here instead: "When the seizures occur between the first month or 40 days and the end of the first full year of life, they are always caused by lack of flow in the five vessels and by failure to complete the patterning of the bones. It can also be caused by lack of breastfeeding and being struck by wind evil."

論曰:

（六）病發身軟，時醒者，謂之癇也。身強直，反張如弓，不時醒者，謂之痓也。

（七）諸反張，大人脊下容側手，小兒容三指者，不可復治也。

（八）凡脈浮之與沉，以判其病在陰陽表裡耳。其浮沉復有大小、滑澀、虛實、遲駃。諸証各依脈形為治。

Commentary III.2 ▻ Brenda Hood

The Gallbladder is an interesting but poorly understood organ. In *Líng Shū* 2, it is described as the palace of central essence (*zhōng jīng zhī fǔ* 中精之府); while *Sù Wèn* 25 states that it arrives when Earth gains Wood (*tǔ dé mù ér dá* 土得木而達), a reference to the idea that Earth moves because of the actions of Wood. The Gallbladder is related to timidity (as seen by the fact that when the Gallbladder is cold one is shy and timid) but also to bones. The Gallbladder's relationship to bones is both via the Foot Shàoyáng Gallbladder channel as well as in its function as an organ. All of the yáng channels of the body affect a particular vital substance and the Foot Shàoyáng Gallbladder channel is said to affect the bones. Most commentators imply that the connection is via the joints as demonstrated by the fact that the joints become disordered when the Foot Shàoyáng channel is diseased. Nevertheless, when long term unresolved fright affects the Gallbladder, the bones become soft. The observation in the present quote that "the bones are timid and incomplete" implies that the yáng aspect of Wood has been adversely affected. Wood is the element/phase of generation (obviously important in an infant) as well as the element/phase related to wind, of which seizures and tetany are manifestations.

III.1 Essay

Line III.1.1 Causes and Forms of Seizures, cont.

(6) If the body during outbreaks goes limp and the patient regains consciousness regularly, we call it "seizures." If the body turns rigid and straight,[5] is arched backwards like a bow, and the patient regains consciousness irregularly, we call it "tetany."

(7) In all cases of arched-back rigidity, if there is a space large enough to place a hand sideways underneath the spine in adults and three fingers in small children, you will not be able to turn the condition around with treatment.[6]

(8) In all cases, [discern] whether the pulse is floating or sunken to determine whether the disease is located in yīn or yáng and in the exterior or interior. [In addition to] this floating or sunken quality [of the pulse], further [discriminate] whether it is large or small, slippery or rough, vacuous or replete, and slow or rapid. Treat the various patterns in each case in accordance with the form of the pulse.

---

5 The *Sūn Zhēn Rén* edition has here: "If the body becomes affected by *kuāng* mania and becomes rigid and straight..."

6 In other words, the outcome will be fatal.

《神農本草經》說

（一）小兒驚癇有一百二十種，其証候微異於常，便是癇候也。

（二）初出腹，血脈不斂，五臟未成，稍將養失宜，即為病也，時不成人。

（三）其經變蒸之後有病，餘証並寬，惟中風最暴卒也。

（四）小兒四肢不好驚掣，氣息小異，欲作癇，及變蒸日滿不解者，並宜龍膽湯也。

（八）凡脈浮之與沉，以判其病在陰陽表裡耳。其浮沉復有大小、滑澀、虛實、遲駛。諸証各依脈形為治。

Commentary III.3 ▻ Brenda Hood

Fright and fear are very different emotions in Chinese medicine. When one is fearful the qì moves down. Anyone who has ever been in a fearful situation can attest to this when they have involuntarily voided themselves. Fright, on the other hand, results in a scattering of qì, something an infant in the process of accumulating and "drawing in" resources for growth can ill afford.

III.1 Essay

Line III.1.2 Quotation from the *Shén Nóng Běn Cǎo Jīng*[1]

(1) There are 120 types of fright seizures[2] in small children. Their signs and symptoms are only slightly different from a normal state of health, but they are nevertheless the signs of seizures.

(2) When babies first emerge from [the mother's] abdomen, the blood vessels fail to draw in and the five *zàng* organs are not yet matured. [At this point, even] slightly inappropriate care and nurturance immediately causes disease. Frequently, [such babies] will not reach adulthood.

(3) If it is after they have passed through the transformations and steamings that they have this disease, all the other residual signs lessen in severity, and it is only wind strike that leads to the most sudden of deaths.

(4) When small children [suffer from] poor health in the four limbs, with fright tugging, shallow and abnormal breathing, imminent seizures, and steamings and transformations that have lasted beyond the full number of days without resolving, Lóngdǎn Tāng is suitable.[3]

---

1 The *Shén Nóng Běn Cǎo Jīng*《神農本草經》("Divine Farmer's Classic of Materia Medica) is an important Hàn dynasty classic that describes 365 medicinal substances by their thermal quality, flavor, and effects on the body, categorizing them into three ranks associated with heaven, humanity, and earth.

2 See Commentary III.3

3 For the formula, see below, pp.51-53.

（一）凡小兒之癇有三種：有風癇，有驚癇，有食癇。

（二）然風癇、驚癇時時有耳，十人之中，未有一二是食癇者。

（三）凡是先寒後熱發者，皆是食癇也。

（四）驚癇當按圖灸之；風癇當與豬心湯；食癇當下乃愈，紫丸佳。

（五）凡小兒所以得風癇者，緣衣暖汗出，風因入也。風癇者，初得之時，先屈指如數，乃發作者。此風癇也。

（六）驚癇者，起於驚怖大啼，乃發作者，此驚癇也。驚癇微者，急持之，勿復更驚之，或自止也。

（七）其先不哺乳，吐而變熱後發癇，此食癇。早下則瘥。

（八）四味紫丸，逐癖飲最良，去病速而不虛人。赤丸瘥快，病重者當用之。

Commentary III.4 ▹ Sabine Wilms

As in many other instances in this book but particularly in the context of the effects of a medicinal preparation, the character *xià* 下 here refers to the therapeutic action of expelling a pathological substance by moving it downward and out of the body. In the context of food seizures, this makes perfect sense since they are the result of the presence of a pathogenic substance in the newborn, contracted through the mother even before birth (see below), or of food accumulations in the body, due to incomplete digestion and failure to disperse ingested food. Wiseman translates the character in this context as "precipitation."

III.1 Essay

Line III.1.3 The Three Types of Seizures

(1) Whenever small children have seizures, there are three types: wind seizures, fright seizures, and food seizures.

(2) This being said, wind seizures and fright seizures are very common but out of ten cases, not even one or two are food seizures.

(3) Whenever you see cold first and then an outbreak of heat, this is always a case of food seizures.

(4) In cases of fright seizures, apply moxibustion according to the [moxibustion] diagrams.[1] For wind seizures, administer Zhūxīn Tāng.[2] For food seizures, induce a downward movement[3] and the patient will recover. Zǐ Wán[4] is excellent [for this purpose].

(5) Whenever small children contract wind seizures, the reason for this is always that they are dressed [too] warmly and sweat, as the result of which wind enters. In cases of wind seizures, when they are initially contracted, the condition first manifests with [the patient's] fingers bending as if they were counting, which is followed by [full-blown] seizures. These are wind seizures.

---

1 It is not clear whether *tú* 圖 ("diagram") here refers a specific illustration or set of illustrations that may have been attached to this text originally or whether it is just a general reference to such charts, examples of which have been found for example among the Dūnhuáng medical manuscripts. For more information on moxibustion charts discovered there, see Vivienne Lo, "Quick and Easy Chinese Medicine: The Dunhuang Moxibustion Charts," (V. Lo and Christopher Cullen, eds., *Medieval Chinese Medicine: The Dunhuang Medical Manuscripts*, Routledge Curzon, 2005.).

2 Zhūxīn Tāng 豬心湯 (Pig Heart Decoction) seems to refer here simply to a soup made from pig hearts, and in that case should probably be translated as "Pig Heart Soup" rather than "Decoction." No other formula for Zhūxīn Tāng is found in the *Qiān Jīn Fāng*.

3 See Commentary III.4

4 For the formula for Zǐ Wán 紫丸 (Purple Pill), see chapter 1 above, pp. 34-35

（一）凡小兒之癇有三種：有風癇，有驚癇，有食癇。

（二）然風癇、驚癇時時有耳，十人之中，未有一二是食癇者。

（三）凡是先寒後熱發者，皆是食癇也。

（四）驚癇當按圖灸之；風癇當與豬心湯；食癇當下乃愈，紫丸佳。

（五）凡小兒所以得風癇者，緣衣暖汗出，風因入也。風癇者，初得之時，先屈指如數，乃發作者。此風癇也。

（六）驚癇者，起於驚怖大啼，乃發作者，此驚癇也。驚癇微者，急持之，勿復更驚之，或自止也。

（七）其先不哺乳，吐而變熱後發癇，此食癇。早下則瘥。

（八）四味紫丸，逐癖飲最良，去病速而不虛人。赤丸瘥快，病重者當用之。

III.1 Essay

Line III.1.3 The Three Types of Seizures, cont.

(6) As for fright seizures, these begin with [the patient] crying loudly after being startled and frightened, after which the seizures occur. These are fright seizures. When fright seizures are [still] slight, hold [the baby] in a tight grip and do not let them be frightened again. It is possible that [the seizures] will stop on their own.

(7) If babies vomit without having been nursed or fed beforehand and then turn hot and afterwards have seizures, these are food seizures. If you induce a downward movement in the early stages [of this disease], recovery will ensue.

(8) Sì Wèi Zǐ Wán[5] and Zhú Pǐ Yǐn[6] are best. They get rid of the disease quickly but do not make the patient empty. Chì Wán[7] causes recovery rapidly and should be used in critical conditions.

---

5 Sì Wèi Zǐ Wán 四味紫丸: Literally, "Four Ingredients Purple Pill," this name almost certainly refers to the formula for Zǐ Wán quoted in Chapter One above, where fright seizures is in fact listed as one of its indications. See pp. 34-38 above.
6 Zhú Pǐ Yǐn 逐癖飲: Literally, "Aggregations-Expelling Drink." I have been unable to find any information on this formula. It could therefore be a generic name for any fluid preparations that have the effect of "expelling aggregations."
7 Literally translated, Chì Wán 赤丸 simply means "Red Pill." There is no formula with this name to be found in this chapter or in the various other contemporary formularies. Nevertheless, as often-cited commentary, presumably by the Sòng editors of the *Qiān Jīn Fāng*, on this important essay points out, the first formula in the chapter below on "Aggregations, Bindings, Distention, and Fullness," namely the formula with eight ingredients called Zǐ Shuāng Wán 紫雙丸 (Double Purple Pill), is red in color because of its use of *zhūshā*. It includes the ingredients *bādòu* and *gānsuì* and should therefore be faster-acting than Zǐ Wán. In accordance with the advice here to administer Chì Wán when Sì Wèi Zǐ Wán is unable to induce a downward movement, and the statement that Chì Wán causes a rapid recovery and should be used in critical conditions, it is possible that the Chì Wán mentioned here is a reference to this formula.

（一）凡小兒不能乳哺，當與紫丸下之。

（二）小兒始生，生氣尚盛。但有微惡，則須下之，必無所損，及其愈病則致深益。

（三）若不時下，則成大疾，疾成則難治矣。

（四）凡下，四味紫丸最善，雖不損人，足以去疾。

（五）若四味紫丸不得下者，當以赤丸下之。赤丸不下，當倍之。

（六）若已下而有餘熱不盡，當按方作龍膽湯，稍稍服之，並摩赤膏。

Commentary III.5 ▹ Sabine Wilms

The concept of "birth qì" (*shēng qì* 生氣) is fascinating to contemplate. I have consciously avoided the more elegant translation of "vital qì," a phrase we commonly encounter in much contemporary Chinese medicine literature in English, because the particular combination of characters suggests something quite different from our customary use of that term. Here it must be referring to a particular qì that perhaps protects or strengthens the baby during the traumatic process of birth and in the most vulnerable time immediately afterwards, but disappears as the newborn enters more firmly into the corporeal body. Alternatively, the term can be interpreted as "generative qì."

III.1 Essay

Line III.1.4 Treating Food Seizures

(1) Whenever small children are unable to nurse or ingest other food, administer Zǐ Wán to cause a downward movement.[1]

(2) Right after babies are born, their birth qì[2] is still exuberant. Nevertheless, if they do have some minor malignity, you must move it down [and out]. [In the course of this treatment,] you must not injure them in any way, and their recovery from the disease will thereby obtain the deepest benefit.

(3) If you fail to move [the illness] downward in time, it will mature into a major illness, and once that illness has matured, it will be difficult to treat indeed!

(4) Whenever you induce a downward movement, Sì Wèi Zǐ Wán is most excellent. Even though it does not injure the patient, it is sufficiently [strong] to get rid of the illness.

(5) If Sì Wèi Zǐ Wán is unable to induce a downward movement, use Chì Wán to move [the illness] downward. If Chì Wán fails to move it downward, double the dosage.

(6) If you have already induced a downward movement and there is still some heat remaining [in the body], prepare Lóngdǎn Tāng according to the formula[3] and administer it in very small doses. At the same time, massage [the patient with] Chì Gāo.[4]

---

1 Literally, the Chinese says, "to move it down," but unfortunately does not specify what is referred to as "it" (*zhī* 之). It is clear from various statements regarding the intended effect of Zǐ Wán, as well as from the constellation of ingredients, that it is aimed at inducing a bowel movement, to eliminate any malign substance that is preventing the intake of additional food by the baby and is the root cause of food seizures. The following line suggests that this may refer to a "minor malignancy" (*wēi è* 微惡), possibly contracted from the mother's incautious diet while still in utero.

2 See Commentary III.5

3 For the formula for Lóngdǎn Tāng, see below pp. 151-153

4 The *Sūn Zhēn Rén* edition here has Shēng Gāo 生膏 (Raw/Fresh Salve) instead. For the formula for Chì Gāo 赤膏 (Red Salve), see the end of this chapter, p. 197.

（一）風癇亦當下之。然當以豬心湯下之。

（二）驚癇但按圖灸之，及摩生膏。不可大下也，何者？驚癇心氣不定，下之內虛益令甚爾。

（三）驚癇甚者，特為難治。故養小兒常慎驚。

（四）勿令聞大聲，抱持之間當安徐，勿令驚怖。

（五）又天雷時，當塞兒耳，並作餘細聲以亂之也。

III.1 Essay

Line III.1.5 Treating Wind and Fright Seizures

(1) Regarding wind seizures, also [treat them by] moving them downward. Nevertheless, in such cases use Zhūxīn Tāng to move them downward.

(2) As for fright seizures, merely treat the patient with moxibustion according to the diagrams[1] and massage with Shēng Gāo. [In patients with fright seizures,] you cannot induce a major downward movement. Why is that? In fright seizures, the heart qì is not settled[2], and if you [treat the patient by] inducing a downward movement, the internal vacuity will be increased even more.

(3) If fright seizures are severe, they are particularly difficult to treat. Therefore constantly beware of fright while rearing small children!

(4) Do not let them hear loud noises and, when holding them in your arms, be still and gentle. Do not let them be frightened or startled!

(5) Moreover, when there is thunder in the sky, plug the children's ears and at the same time make some other subtle noises in order to distract them.

---

1 For more information on moxibustion charts, see note 1 to line III.1.3, p. 117 above.

2 Another edition has *zú* 足 ("sufficient") instead of *dìng* 定 ("settled.")

（一）凡養小兒，皆微驚以長其血脈，但不欲大驚。

（二）大驚乃灸驚脈。

（三）若五六十日灸者，驚復更甚，生百日後灸驚脈乃善。

（四）兒有熱，不欲哺乳，臥不安，又數驚，此癇之初也。服紫丸便愈。不愈復與之。

（五）兒眠時小驚者，一月輒一以紫丸下之，減其盛氣，令兒不病癇也。

Commentary III.6 ▻ Sabine Wilms

Jīng mài 驚脈: This compound is not a standard medical term transmitted in other classical texts. My best guess is that it is simply a reference to the specific vessels, or more specifically the points thereon, that were commonly used to treat fright in small children with moxibustion. Similar to the general reference to moxibustion charts above, this generic statement here seems to suggest that this information was so common and widely available that there was no need for Sūn Sīmiǎo to take up precious space to repeat it here. Unfortunately, such charts have not been preserved as part of any existing versions of the *Qiān Jīn Fāng* or any other pediatric literature. For another example of treating fright by manipulating the qì in certain channels, in this case by acupuncture, see *Sù Wèn* 28: 刺痫惊脉五，针手太阴各五，刺经太阳五，刺手少阴经络傍者一，足阳明一，上踝五寸刺三针 ("Needle seizures with fright in the vessels in five places: Needle the hand's Tàiyīn in five times each, needle the Tàiyáng channel five times, needle once to the side of the hand's Shàoyīn channels and network vessels, needle once on the foot's Yángmíng, and needle three times by the ankle, five *cùn* above.").

III.1 Essay

Line III.1.6 Treating Fright with Moxibustion or Zǐ Wán

(1) Whenever you are rearing small children, always expose them to mild fright, in order to lengthen their blood vessels, but you do not want to expose them to great fright.

(2) [If they have been exposed to] great fright, apply moxibustion to the fright vessels.[1]

(3) If you have [treated them with] moxibustion [at the age of] 50 or 60 days [after birth] and they get frightened again even more severely, it is excellent to apply moxibustion on the fright vessels a hundred days after birth.

(4) If children have heat [in their body], do not want to nurse or be fed, are sleeping restlessly, and have furthermore been exposed to fright repeatedly, this is the beginning of seizures! Administer Zǐ Wán to induce recovery. If they fail to recover, give it again.

(5) If children [have been exposed] to minor fright while sleeping, give Zǐ Wán once a month to induce a downward movement. This will reduce their exuberant qì and keep the child from [contracting] the disease of seizures.

---

1 See Commentary III.6

（一）兒立夏後有病，治之慎勿妄灸，不欲吐下。

（二）但以除熱湯浴之，除熱散粉之，除熱赤膏摩之，又以膏塗臍中。

（三）令兒在涼處，勿禁水漿，常以新水飲之。

III.1 Essay

Line III.1.7 Treatment in the Summer

(1) If children contract a disease after the Beginning of Summer,[1] when you treat them, beware! Do not recklessly apply moxibustion, and do not induce vomiting or a downward movement [either]!

(2) Only bathe them with heat-eliminating decoctions, sprinkle heat-eliminating powders on them, and massage them with heat-eliminating red salve.[2] Furthermore, apply the salve to the center of the navel.

(3) Keep the child in a cool location, do not restrict intake of water and thick liquids, and constantly give them fresh water to drink.

---

1 *Lì xià* 立夏: This is one of the 24 seasonal markers, known as *jié qì* 節氣, literally "nodal qì" or solar terms. It is the reference to a specific date that always falls around the sixth day of the fifth lunar month.

2 For a variety of formulas for heat-eliminating decoctions and powders, see Chapter Five on Cold Damage forthcoming in Part Two of this translation series of Sūn Sīmiǎo's writings on pediatrics. Since there is no specific formula for a "Red Salve" mentioned in that chapter, this last instruction to use "heat-eliminating red salve" is most likely a reference to the formula for Dānshēn Chì Gāo (Red Salvia Salve), given in line III.4.1 below on p. 197.

（一）小兒衣甚薄，則腹中乳食不消，不消則大便皆醋臭，此欲為癖之漸。

（二）便將紫丸以微消之。

（三）服法：先從少起，常令大便稀，勿大下也。

（四）稀後便漸減之，不醋臭乃止藥也。

Commentary III.7 ▻ Sabine Wilms

Rǔ shí bù xiāo 乳食不消: I have chosen to translate the character *xiāo* 消 literally in this expression because its meaning is more specific than the English term "to digest." Marked by the water radical, it means "to vanish," "to melt away," or "to be used up." In the *Shuō Wén Jiě Zì*, it is glossed as *jìn* 盡, "to exhaust" or "use up to the end." In the context of digesting food, it refers to the failure of the digestive system to break up ingested food. This dysfunction has the following results: Instead of dispersing, the ingested food remains in the abdomen for a prolonged period of time, blocking flow and rotting instead of being digested. It is then either eliminated as foul-smelling feces or, in a more serious development, forms pathological masses in the abdominal area. At the same time, the child is unable to absorb the nutrients in the food and ends up being deprived of necessary nutrition.

III.1 Essay

Line III.1.8 Treatment of Aggregations

(1) When small children are dressed in very thin clothes, the milk and [other] food in their abdomen fail to disperse.[1] When [the milk and food] do not disperse, the stools all [become] sour and foul-smelling. This means that they are about to suffer from a gradual development of aggregations.[2]

(2) In that case, give Zǐ Wán to subtly disperse them.[3]

(3) Method of administration: First begin with small amounts, which you give constantly until you have caused the stools to become runny. Do not induce a great downward movement!

(4) After [the stools] have become runny, gradually reduce [the dosage]. When [the stools] are no longer sour and foul-smelling, then [you can] stop the medicine.

Commentary III.8 ▻ Sabine Wilms

Pǐ 癖: This term refers to a condition that is explained in the *Zhū Bìng Yuán Hòu Lùn* as follows: "Blockage in the *sānjiāo* results in a lack of free flow in the intestines and stomach. Because the person has drunk too much water and thick liquids, cold lodges and stagnates instead of dispersing. If the person then encounters cold qì, it accumulates and forms aggregations. 'Aggregations' refers to [accumulations that are located] off to the side in the space of both rib-sides, sometimes manifesting with pain." See *Zhū Bìng Yuán Hòu Lùn*, volume 20, entry on "Aggregations."

1 See Commentary III.7

2 See Commentary III.8

3 Due to the vagueness of classical Chinese grammar, *zhī* 之 can refer either to the milk and food or to the aggregations. I have consciously chosen a translation that leaves the choice up to the reader, but given the etiology of this disease, this doesn't make a difference anyway since the aggregations form out of undispersed food and breast milk.

（一）凡小兒冬月下無所畏，夏月下難瘥。

（二）然有病者，不可不下，下後腹中當小脹滿，故當節哺乳數日，不可妄下。

（三）又乳哺小兒，常令多少有常劑，兒漸大，當稍稍增之。

（四）若減少者，此腹中已有小不調也。便微服藥，勿復哺之，但當與乳。甚者十數日，微者五六日止，哺自當如常。

III.1 Essay

Line III.1.9a Importance of Early Treatment

(1) In all cases of treating small children, when you induce downward movement[1] in the winter months, there is nothing to fear.[2] When you induce downward movement in the summer months, however, it is difficult for them to recover.

(2) Nevertheless, if the patient has a disease, you [may] have no choice but to [treat it by] down-moving. After you have moved [the disease] down, there should be minor distention and fullness in the center of the abdomen. Therefore you must moderate feeding and nursing for several days. You must not recklessly induce downward movement!

(3) Furthermore, in nursing and feeding small children, always dose the amount consistently! As babies gradually grow bigger, you can increase it little by little.

(4) If [their food intake] is reduced, this means that they already have a minor disharmony in the abdomen. In that case, administer mild medicinal preparations. Do not feed anything else but give only breast milk! In severe cases, [follow this advice] for more than ten days; in mild cases, you can stop after five or six days. Then you can resume feeding as usual.

---

1 Literally, the text simply says "In all cases of downward movement in small children..." Based on context, however, it is clear that this phrase is not referring here to naturally occurring diarrhea but to bowel movements that are the result of medical treatment, for the purposes mentioned above of clearing heat, fright, or other pathogens.

2 The *Huá Xià* edition of the *Qiān Jīn Fāng* here has *wú suǒ wèi* 無所謂, which changes the meaning of this phrase a bit from "there is nothing to fear" to "there is nothing to talk about," in the sense of "it doesn't matter."

（一）若都不肯食哺，而但欲乳者，此是有癖。

（二）為疾重，要當下之，不可不下。

（三）不下則致寒熱或吐而發癇，或更致下痢。

（四）此皆病重，不早下之所為也，此即難治矣。

（五）但先治其輕時，兒不耗損而病速愈矣。

Commentary III.9 ▻ Sabine Wilms

I follow Nigel Wiseman in translating *lì* 痢 as "dysentery" here, in the sense explained in the *Practical Dictionary of Chinese Medicine*, p. 163, as "a disease characterized by abdominal pain, tenesmus, and stool containing pus and blood." While the character 痢 is sometimes used interchangeably with 利 (denoting "disinhibition" or in the context of stools, just "diarrhea") in early texts, the specific context here suggests a more severe pathology that would warrant the conscious choice of the stronger term 痢. While the English term "dysentery" now suggests the biomedical connotation of an infection, specifically by Shigella bacteria or by the ameba Entamoeba histolytica, the term dysentery has historically been defined in English as severe diarrhea with tenesmus, pain, and passage of mucus and blood in the feces.

III.1 Essay

Line III.1.9b Importance of Early Treatment

(1) If they are completely unwilling to eat anything at all that you are trying to feed them but only want to nurse, this means the presence of aggregations.

(2) This means that it is urgent and critical, and you want to [treat by] inducing a downward movement. You have no choice but to [treat such conditions by] inducing a downward movement!

(3) If you do not induce a downward movement, [such conditions] will lead to cold and heat, possibly vomiting, and then the outbreak of seizures. It will possibly even lead to dysentery.[1]

(4) All of these [outcomes] are critical conditions that are due to the fact that you did not move [the disease] down in the early stages. These conditions are then difficult to treat!

(5) If you had only treated [the disease earlier] at a stage when it was still mild, the child would not have suffered such harm but would have recovered quickly from the disease!

---

1 See Commentary III.9

（一）凡小兒屎黃而臭者，此腹中有伏熱。宜微將服龍膽湯。

（二）若白而醋者，此挾宿食不消也。當服紫丸。

（三）微者少與藥，令內消。 甚者小增藥，令小下。

（四）皆復節乳哺數日，令胃氣平和。

（五）若不節乳哺，則病易復。復下之則傷其胃氣，令腹脹滿。

（六）再三下之尚可，過則傷矣。

III.1 Essay

Line III.1.10 Latent Heat in the Abdomen

(1) Whenever small children have yellow foul-smelling stools, this means the presence of latent heat in the abdomen. It is appropriate to administer Lóngdǎn Tāng with subtlety.

(2) If the stools are white and sour-smelling, this means that the condition is complicated by abiding food that is failing to disperse. [In such cases,] administer Zǐ Wán.

(3) In minor cases, give just a scant amount of medicine to cause [the abiding food] to disperse internally. In severe cases, slightly increase the medicine to induce a minor downward movement.

(4) In both situations, again moderate nursing and feeding for several days to allow the stomach qì to become even and harmonious.

(5) If you do not moderate nursing and feeding, the disease will easily return. If you then again [treat it by] down-moving, you damage [the patient]'s stomach qì, causing abdominal distention and fullness.

(6) [Treating the patient] up to three times by inducing downward movements may still be permissible, but if you exceed this number, damage results!

（一）凡小兒有癖，其脈大必發癇，此為食癇。下之便愈。

（二）當審候掌中與三指脈，不可令起。

（三）而不時下，致於發癇，則難療矣。

（四）若早下之，此脈終不起也。

（五）脈在掌中尚可早療，若至指則病增矣。

（一）凡小兒腹中有疾生，則身寒熱。寒熱則血脈動，動則心不定。

（二）心不定則易驚，驚則癇發速也。

III.1 Essay

Line III.1.11 Preventing Aggregations from Turning into Food Seizures

(1) In all cases of small children suffering from aggregations, if their vessels are large,[1] an outbreak of seizures is bound to occur. This is [the disease] of food seizures. Moving [the aggregations] downward will cure the patient.

(2) Examine [the patient's hand] for a vessel from the center of the palm into the middle finger.[2] You cannot allow [this vessel] to rise [from the palm of the hand into the finger].

(3) If you do not move [the aggregation] down in time, this will lead to the outbreak of seizures. As a result, the condition will be difficult to cure!

(4) If you had moved it down early on, this vessel would have ended instead of rising [into the finger].

(5) If the vessel is still in the center of the palm, [this means that you] can still cure [the disease] in this early stage. If it has reached the finger, the disease has increased [in severity]!

Line III.1.12 Instability of the Heart

(1) In all cases of small children suffering from any illnesses forming in the abdomen, generalized cold and heat result. As the result of the cold and heat, the blood stirs in the vessels, and as the result of this stirring, there is instability in the heart.

(2) Instability of the heart then results in a tendency to contract fright, and the fright then results in the speedy outbreak of seizures.

---

1 My translation of *mài* 脈 as "vessel" here instead of as "pulse" --in which case it would be translated as "if their pulse is large"-- is based on the paragraph below on "Diagnosing Seizures" (line III.2.1), where the term clearly refers to the vessel since its color is described as a diagnostic sign. While the difference between "vessel" and "pulse" sounds important in English, it is ultimately perhaps not that critical in the context of Chinese medicine since a large pulse, or in other words, flow in the vessel, is merely an indication of a large vessel.

2 Alternatively, *sān zhǐ mài* 三指脈 can also be read as a technical term referring to a method of palpitation where all three fingers are used, i.e., at the *cùn* 寸, *guān* 關, and *chǐ* 尺 positions. My more literal reading here as "the vessel at the third [i.e., middle] finger" is based on the context of this entire paragraph. In addition, this interpretation is supported by the fact that the radial pulse position is so small in an infant that it may be difficult to read.

（一）夫癇，小兒之惡病也，或有不及求醫而致困者也。

（二）然氣發於內，必先有候。

（三）常宜審察其精神而採其候也。

（一）手白肉魚際脈黑者，是癇候。

（二）魚際脈赤者熱。

（三）脈青大者寒，脈青細為平也。

III.2 Rules for Diagnosing Seizures

Line III.2.1

(1) Now seizures are a malign disease in small children! There is a real possibility that a doctor cannot be consulted in time and that great peril ensues.

(2) Nevertheless, for qì to erupt on the inside, there will necessarily be signs [of it] beforehand.

(3) It is [therefore] recommended that you constantly scrutinize the *jīngshén* and pick out the signs for this [disease].

Line III.2.2

(1) If the vessel in the white flesh of the hand at Yújì[1] is black, this is a sign for seizures.

(2) If the vessel at Yújì is red, it means heat.

(3) If the vessel is green-blue and enlarged, it means cold. If the vessel is green-blue and fine, it means a balanced state.[2]

1 Literally "fish margin," this is a common technical term referring to the middle of the thenar eminence, now known as the modern point LU-10.

2 *Píng* 平 here refers to a normal, healthy state of being, neither too hot nor too cold, as opposed to the enlarged state or abnormal colors of the vessel that indicate seizures or heat or cold.

（一）鼻口乾燥，大小便不利，是癇候。

（二）眼不明，上視喜陽，是癇候。

（三）耳後完骨上有青絡盛，臥不靜，是癇候。青脈刺之，令血出也。

（四）小兒發逆上，啼笑面暗，色不變，是癇候。

（五）鼻口青，時小驚，是癇候。

（六）目閉青，時小驚，是癇候。

III.2 Rules for Diagnosing Seizures

Line III.2.3

(1) If the [child's] nose and mouth are dry, and urination and defecation are inhibited, this is a sign for seizures.

(2) If the eyes are not bright but stare upward and have a preference for yáng,[1] this is a sign for seizures.

(3) The presence of exuberance in the green-blue network vessels behind the ear above Wángǔ,[2] in combination with restless sleep, is a sign for seizures. Needle these green-blue vessels, making them bleed.

(4) If small children suffer outbreaks of counterflow ascent in combination with wailing and laughing[3] and a darkened face with a complexion that does not change, this is a sign for seizures.

(5) A green-blue nose and mouth, accompanied by periodic minor fright, are a sign for seizures.

(6) Eyes that are shut and green-blue, accompanied by periodic minor fright, are a sign for seizures.

---

1 I.e., the child's eyes are dim and stare straight up into the sun instead of avoiding the intensity of sunlight, as healthy babies would do.

2 Literally "completion bone," this is roughly equivalent to the mastoid process and the modern point GB-12.

3 Another edition has *tí kū* 啼哭 ("wailing and crying").

（一）身熱，頭常汗出，是癇候。

（二）身熱，吐哯而喘，是癇候。

（三）身熱，目時直視，是癇候。

（四）臥惕惕而驚，手足振搖，是癇候。

（五）臥夢笑，手足動搖，是癇候。

（一）意氣下而妄怒，是癇候。

（二）咽乳不利，是癇候。

（三）目瞳子卒大黑於常，是癇候。

（四）喜欠，目上視，是癇候。

（五）身熱，小便難，是癇候。

（六）身熱，目視不精，是癇候。

（七）吐痢不止，厥痛時起，是癇候。

（八）弄舌搖頭，是癇候。

III.2 Rules for Diagnosing Seizures

Line III.2.4

(1) Generalized heat with constant sweating from the head is a sign for seizures.

(2) Generalized heat with vomiting and panting is a sign for seizures.

(3) Generalized heat with eyes that periodically stare straight ahead is a sign for seizures.

(4) During sleep, exhibiting great fearfulness and then fright and flailing hands and feet is a sign for seizures.

(5) During sleep, laughing in dreams and flailing hands and feet is a sign for seizures.

Line III.2.5

(1) Belching and descent of qì followed by outbreaks of rash anger is a sign for seizures.

(2) Inhibited swallowing of breast milk is a sign for seizures.

(3) Pupils that are suddenly enlarged and blacker than normal are a sign for seizures.

(4) A tendency to yawning and upward-staring eyes is a sign for seizures.

(5) Generalized heat with difficult urination is a sign for seizures.

(6) Generalized heat with unfocused vision is a sign for seizures.

(7) Incessant vomiting and dysentery with periodically arising reversal pain is a sign for seizures.

(8) Sticking out the tongue and shaking the head is a sign for seizures.

（一）以上諸候二十條，皆癇之初也。

（二）見其候，便抓其陽脈所應灸。

（三）抓之皆重手，令兒驟啼，及足絕脈。亦依方與湯。

（四）直視瞳子動，腹滿轉鳴，下血身熱，口噤不得乳，反張脊強，汗出發熱，為臥不悟，手足掣瘲善驚，凡八條，癇之劇者也。

（五）如有此，非復湯抓所能救，便當時灸。

III.2 Rules for Diagnosing Seizures

Line III.2.6

(1) The various signs in the twenty items above all [indicate] the beginning of seizures.

(2) When you see these signs, scrape[1] the baby's yáng vessels[2] at the place where you should apply moxibustion.

(3) When scraping, always do so with a heavy hand so you make the child cry abruptly, and sufficient[ly strong] to cut off the vessels.[3] Also administer decoctions in accordance with the formulas.

(4) Straight forward-staring eyes with moving pupils; abdominal fullness with churning and rumbling; lower-body bleeding and generalized heat; clenched mouth preventing the baby from nursing; a backward-stretched rigid spine; sweating with heat effusion; failing to wake up from sleep; and tugging and slackening in the hands and feet with a tendency to fright, these eight signs all serve as indications for the acute stage of seizures.

(5) If these are present, the patient can no longer be rescued by means of decoctions or scraping. In such cases, you must treat the patient at that time with moxibustion.

---

1 *Zhuā* 抓: Consisting of the two components "hand" and "claw/nail," this character is generally translated as "to scratch" but here most likely refers to the vigorous rubbing and scraping that is performed as a medical treatment commonly called *guā shā* 刮痧.

2 *Yáng mài* 陽脈: The meaning of this compound is somewhat obscure here, but it could refer to the Yángmíng vessel, as this vessel contains lots of qì and blood, and scraping it would therefore reduce both, or to the Tàiyáng bladder channel on the back, a common location for *guā shā* treatments. As another possibility, the term could refer specifically to the location of Dàzhuī ("Great Hammer," DU-14), the meeting point of all the yáng channels.

3 *Zú jué mài* 足絕脈: This phrase changes meaning drastically, depending on whether you read 足 as "foot" or as "enough." If you interpret it as "foot," the phrase could be then understood as part of the following sentence in the sense of "When the condition has reached the point where the vessel is cut off in the foot,..." One could even argue for an interpretation as "where the pulse has expired in the foot." As indicated by their choice of punctuation, most modern editions appear to follow this line of interpretation. The reason I read 足 as "sufficient" and punctuate as I have done above is an almost literally identical line found in an important pediatric text called *Yòu Yòu Xīn Shū* 《幼幼新書》 ("New Writings About Children", composed by Liú Fǎng 劉昉 in the Sòng dynasty), which reads as follows: 爪之皆重手，令兒驟啼乃絕，亦依方與湯。("When scraping, always use a heavy hand to make the child cry abruptly and cut off [the vessel]. Also give decoctions according to the [proper] formula.").

論曰：

（一）若病家始發便來詣師，師可診候。

（二）所解為法，作次序治之，以其節度首尾取瘥也。

（三）病家已經雜治無次序，不能制病，病則變異其本候後，師便不知其前証虛實，直依其後証作治，亦不得瘥也。

Commentary III.10 ▻ Sabine Wilms

Here, *shī* 師 refers to a high-level practitioner in the sense of the ideal physician described in Sūn Sīmiǎo's chapter on medical ethics in Volume One of the *Qiān Jīn Fāng*. It is interesting to note how Sun Sīmiǎo goes out of his way throughout this essay to avoid blaming any involved physician but squarely assigns responsibility for the failure of medical treatment to the patient's family. Rather than allowing for the possibility that the first physician might have prescribed the wrong medicine, Sūn blames the patient's family for lacking trust in the first physician's approach to treatment and for recklessly consulting a second physician before giving the treatment prescribed by the first one enough time to be effective.

III.3 Essay

Line III.3.1

(1) If, as soon as [fright seizures] erupt, the patient is taken to consult a master [physician],[1] this master will be able to diagnose the signs.

(2) Using an understanding [of the patient's condition on the basis of these first signs], [such a physician] will set up a method and establish the proper sequence in which to administer treatment, thereby obtaining recovery by figuring out head and tail [of the disease] on the basis of the regular progression.

(3) If the patient [however] has already undergone miscellaneous treatments with no regard for the proper sequence, and [the treatments] were unable to control the disease, the disease will then have transformed into a condition that is different from the root signs. A master [who gets involved subsequently] then does not know whether the previous [manifestations of the disease] were evidence for vacuity or repletion. Devising a treatment directly in accordance only with the later evidence, [this master] will therefore not be able to achieve recovery either.

1 See Commentary III.10

論曰：

（一）要應精問察之，為前師所配，依取其前蹤跡以為治，乃無逆耳。

（二）前師處湯，本應數劑乃瘥，而病家服一兩劑未效，便謂不驗，已後更問他師。

（三）師不尋前人為治寒溫次序，而更為治而不次前師，治則弊也。

（四）或前已下之，後須平和療以接之，而得瘥也。

（五）或前人未下之，或不去者，或前治寒溫失度，後人應調治之，是為治敗病，皆須邀射之，然後免耳。

（六）不依次第，及不審察，必及重弊也。

III.3 Essay

Line III.3.2

(1) It is crucial to scrutinize the situation in response to detailed questioning, to match [your actions] to what the previous master did, and to administer treatment in accordance with the traces of the previous [history of this condition]. Only then will you avoid being out of alignment.[1]

(2) When the previous master prescribed a decoction, originally [the patient] should have been cured after several batches. [In this case,] however, the patient took one or two batches, which did not yet deliver any results, then pronounced them to be ineffective, and subsequently went on to consult another master.

(3) If the [newly involved] master fails to follow the previous person's [proper] treatment sequence for cold or heat, but administers treatments without following [the treatment methodology of] the previous master, the treatment will result in harm.

(4) It is possible that the previous treatment has already brought the disease down,[2] [in which case] you must [merely follow up] afterwards by evening out and harmonizing, and you will achieve recovery.

(5) Alternatively, if the previous person either did not yet bring [the disease] down or failed to remove it, or the previous treatment for cold or warmth was inappropriately measured, the subsequent person should treat the patient in attunement [with this specific situation]. This is a case of treating a vanquished disease. In all such cases, you must "track it down to shoot it"[3] and then afterwards avoid it.

(6) If you do not follow the proper sequence and fail to scrutinize [the situation] carefully, you will invariably end up doubling the harm.

---

1 *Nì* 逆 in this context most likely means to act in violation of the natural progression back towards health.

2 Here, *xià* 下 ("moving [the disease] down") is used in the sense of successfully eliminating the disease-causing agent by means of inducing a downward movement in the treatment methodology described in the previous chapter.

3 In the commentary to the Rén Mín Wèi Shēng edition, this expression is paraphrased as "pursuing" (*móu qiú* 謀求), but I prefer the more literal reading.

龍膽湯

（一）治嬰兒出腹，血脈盛實，寒熱溫壯，四肢驚掣，發熱，大吐哯者。

（二）若已能進哺，中食實不消，壯熱。

（三）及變蒸不解，中客人鬼氣，並諸驚癇，方悉主之。

（四）十歲以下小兒皆服之，小兒龍膽湯第一，此是新出腹嬰兒方。

（五）若日月長大者，以次依此為例。

（六）若必知客忤及有魃氣者，可加人參，當歸，各如龍膽多少也。

（七）一百日兒加三銖，二百日兒加六銖，一歲兒加半兩，餘藥皆準耳。

III.4 Lóngdǎn Tāng (Gentian Decoction)

Indications

(1) A formula for babies fresh out of the belly, to treat exuberant repletion in the blood vessels, cold and heat with vigorous warmth, fright with flailing of the four limbs, heat effusion, and severe vomiting.

(2) If [the patient] is already able to ingest food, [this decoction also treats] being struck by food, with repletion, failure to disperse [the food], and vigorous fever.

(3) [The formula is also indicated for] transformations and steamings that fail to resolve, being struck by intrusion by human or ghost qì, as well as the various forms of fright seizures. This formula governs them all completely.

(4) Any small children under the age of ten *suì* can take this [formula]. The reason why Lóngdǎn Tāng is the first [formula] for small children is that it is a formula for babies who have just come out of the belly.

(5) If they are older than that, take [the information] following [the formula instructions here] and rely on this as precedent.

(6) If you know without a doubt that [the patient is suffering from] intrusive upset or the presence of *qí* ghost qì,[1] you can add *rénshēn* and *dāngguī*, each in roughly the same amount as the *lóngdǎn*.

(7) For a 100-day-old child, add 3 *zhū*; for a 200-day-old child, add 6 *zhū*; for a 1-*suì*-old child, add 0.5 *liǎng*. Adjust all the other medicinals accordingly.

---

1 *Qí* 魁 is the name for a special kind of ghosts, namely those of small children. The *Zhū Bìng Yuán Hòu Lùn*, vol. 47, entry on "Possession by Qí Ghosts," explains that the condition is contracted in utero, when the pregnant woman's fetus is possessed by another baby's ghost that has been led into the abdomen by an evil spirit. It manifests with slight diarrhea, intermittent cold and heat, and coarse and lusterless hair.

龍膽湯

龍膽	六銖
鈎藤皮	六銖
柴胡	六銖
黃芩	六銖
桔梗	六銖
芍藥	六銖
茯苓	一方作茯神,六銖
甘草	六銖
蜣螂	二枚,炙
大黃	一兩

（一）上十味，㕮咀，以水一升，煮取五合為劑也。服之如後節度。

（二）藥有虛實，虛藥宜足數合水也。

（三）兒生一日至七日，分一合為三服；兒生八日至十五日，分一合半為三服；生十六日至二十日，分二合為三服；兒生二十日至三十日，分三合為三服；兒生三十日至四十日，盡以五合為三服。

（四）皆得下即止，勿再服也。

III.4 Lóngdǎn Tāng (Gentian Decoction)

Ingredients

lóngdǎn	6 *zhū*
gōuténgpí	6 *zhū*
cháihú	6 *zhū*
huángqín	6 *zhū*
jiégěng	6 *zhū*
sháoyào	6 *zhū*
fúlíng	6 *zhū* (another formula uses *fúshén* instead)
gāncǎo	6 *zhū*
qiāngláng	2 pcs (dry-roasted)
dàhuáng	1 *liǎng*

Preparation

(1) Pound the ten ingredients above and boil in 1 *shēng* of water until reduced to 5 *gě*, to make one batch. To administer [the medicine], measure out the appropriate amount according to the following information.

(2) This medicine can be used for either vacuity or repletion. As a medicine for vacuity, just using several *gě* of water is sufficient.

(3) For a child born in the past one to seven days, divide 1 *gě* into three doses. For a child born in the past eight to fifteen days, divide 1.5 *gě* into three doses. For a child born in the past sixteen to twenty days, divide 2 *gě* into three doses. For a child born in the past twenty to thirty days, divide 3 *gě* into three doses. For a child born in the past thirty to forty days, use the full 5 *gě*, administered in three doses.

(4) In all cases, stop immediately when you have achieved a downward movement. Do not give any further doses.

龍膽湯《千金要方衍義》

（一）紫丸，治初生小兒痰癖內結；龍膽湯，治初生小兒血脈實盛。

（二）原其痰癖，良因母氣虛寒，乳哺不化而結。

（三）詳其實盛，多緣母之嗜慾不節，毒遺胎息而熱。

（四）殊非稟氣之充，血脈有餘之謂。蓋結非熱不散，實非寒不解。

（五）龍膽苦寒，專去肝旺實熱。鉤藤、柴胡、黃芩、芍藥皆清理二家之匡佐。蜣蜋一味，方中罕用，考之《本經》為小兒驚癇瘛瘲之專藥，為藥中健卒，得大黃為內應，何憚彈丸不克耶。茯苓、甘草用以留中，安輯邦畿，尤不可缺。

（六）此與紫丸分途異治，功力並馳。

Lóngdǎn Tāng (Gentian Decoction) *Yǎn Yì* (Expanded Meaning)

(1) Zǐ Wán[1] treats phlegm aggregations binding internally in newborn babies, while Lóngdǎn Tāng treats repletion and exuberance in the blood vessels in newborn babies.

(2) As for the origin of phlegm aggregations, they are reliably caused by vacuity cold in the mother's qì, as a result of which the breast milk that the baby has consumed fails to transform but binds instead.

(3) Taking a close look at the fullness and exuberance [in the blood vessels that is the root cause addressed by Lóngdǎn Tāng], in most cases this is caused by the mother's failure to reign in her cravings. The poison was transmitted to the fetus where it increased in severity and turned into heat.

(4) To be specific, [this fullness and exuberance in the blood vessels] is not a case of constitutional qì being too ample and there being an overabundance in the blood vessels. Thus, the [internal] binding [of the phlegm aggregations that is addressed by Zǐ Wán] is not a case of heat failing to disperse, and the repletion is not a case of cold failing to resolve.

1 For the formula and discussion of Zǐ Wán, see chapter 1, pages 33-41

龍膽湯《千金要方衍義》

（一）紫丸，治初生小兒痰澼內結；龍膽湯，治初生小兒血脈實盛。

（二）原其痰澼，良因母氣虛寒，乳哺不化而結。

（三）詳其實盛，多緣母之嗜慾不節，毒遺胎息而熱。

（四）殊非稟氣之充，血脈有餘之謂。蓋結非熱不散，實非寒不解。

（五）龍膽苦寒，專去肝旺實熱。鉤藤、柴胡、黃芩、芍藥皆清理二家之匡佐。蜣蜋一味，方中罕用，考之《本經》為小兒驚癇瘛瘲之專藥，為藥中健卒，得大黃為內應，何憚彈丸不克耶。茯苓、甘草用以留中，安輯邦畿，尤不可缺。

（六）此與紫丸分途異治，功力並馳。

Lóngdǎn Tāng (Gentian Decoction) *Yǎn Yì* (Expanded Meaning), cont.

(5) *Lóngdǎn* is bitter and cold and specifically gets rid of liver effulgence with repletion heat. *Gōuténg, cháihú, huángqín,* and *sháoyào* are all assistants in the two categories of clearing and regulating medicinals. The single ingredient *qiāngláng* is rarely used in formulas. When I researched it in the *Shén Nóng Běn Cǎo Jīng,*[2] [I learned that] it is a medicinal specifically used for small children's fright seizures with tugging and slackening. It acts as a vigorous foot soldier in this medicine and as the internal correspondent to *dàhuáng*. How could you fear that its ammunition will not overcome [the enemy][3]? *Fúlíng* and *gāncǎo* are used to retain the center and to "pacify the territory." [These two ingredients] are particularly indispensable.

(6) Lóngdǎn Tāng and Zǐ Wán go their separate ways to provide different treatments, but their efficacy and strength are equally swift.

2 The *Shén Nóng Běn Cǎo Jīng* 《神農本草經》 is an anonymous text that was compiled in the Hàn period. Literally translated, the title means "Divine Farmer's Classic of Materia Medica." In Chinese medical literature, it is commonly abbreviated as *Běn Jīng* 本經. It is the earliest extant text of Chinese pharmaceutical knowledge that continues to be cited to this day. It records information on 365 medicinal substances, which are classified into three grades in relation to their medicinal efficacy (*dú* 毒).

3 My interpretation of this last phrase is simply my best guess. While *dàn wán* 彈丸 can just refer to pellet-shaped ammunition, such as that used for slingshots or catapults, it is also commonly used to describe the balls formed from fecal matter by the dung beetles to store their food in. The line could then mean "How could you not overcome your dread of dung balls [given the medicinal benefits of this ingredient]?" Nevertheless, as a medicinal ingredient, the whole body of the dung beetle is used, not the pellets produced by the living insect. Since the formula discussed here is for a decoction, it cannot be a reference to the pills that include *qiāngláng* as an ingredient either. Thus reading this phrase as something like "How could you fear that these pills [that are described in the formula discussed in this line] would be unable to conquer [the disease]?" seems unlikely. Given the frequent use of military analogies in the *Qiān Jīn Fāng Yǎn Yì*, I have chosen to simply read *dàn wán* as "ammunition."

大黃湯

治少小風癇積聚，腹痛夭矯，二十五癇方。

大黃	三銖
人參	三銖
細辛	三銖
乾薑	三銖
當歸	三銖
甘皮	三銖

上六味，㕮咀，以水一升，煮取四合。服之如許，日三。

III.5 Dàhuáng Tāng (Rhubarb Decoction)

Indications

A formula that treats wind seizures in early childhood, with accumulations and gatherings and abdominal pain so bad that it makes the patient bend and twist, as well as the twenty-five [forms of] seizures.

Ingredients

dàhuáng	3 *zhū*
rénshēn	3 *zhū*
xìxīn	3 *zhū*
gānjiāng	3 *zhū*
dāngguī	3 *zhū*
gānpí	3 *zhū*

Preparation

Pound the six ingredients above and decoct in 1 *shēng* of water until reduced to 4 *gě*. Take an amount roughly the size of a jujube, three times a day.

大黃湯《千金要方衍義》

（一）方下所治少小風癇，明是木邪內盛，乘克中土。殊非外風襲入之謂。

（二）故於理中方內除去白朮之滯、甘草之緩，但取參、薑，參入細辛以散內盛之風。

（三）當歸以調紊亂之血，甘皮以豁壅遏之痰，大黃以滌固結之積。

（四）與黃龍湯同一手筆。彼以病氣盤錯，胃氣傷殘，雖用硝黃徒增脹滿，必藉人參大力，以鼓盪綀之威。

（五）此以孩提血氣未實，不勝病氣留連，雖宜大黃迅掃，必兼參、薑溫散，可無傷中之虞。

（六）然此僅堪為智者道，難使庸俗知也。

Dàhuáng Tāng (Rhubarb Decoction) *Yǎn Yì* (Expanded Meaning)

(1) The wind seizures in early childhood that this formula treats are clearly a case of internal exuberance of wood evil that is overwhelming center earth. To be specific, [this formula] does not address an invasion of wind from the outside.

(2) For this reason, [the current formula] has removed the stagnating action of *báizhú* and the moderating action of *gāncǎo* from the Lǐ Zhōng formula family,[1] but has chosen *rénshēn* and *gānjiāng* [from that formula] to join hands with *xìxīn* to disperse the internally exuberant wind.

(3) *Dāngguī* is used to attune the chaotically moving blood, *gānpí* to split apart the congesting phlegm, and *dàhuáng* to flush out the solidified and bound gatherings.

1 *Lǐ Zhōng* 理中, literally "Center-Regulating," is a well-known group of formulas going back to the decoction with this name in the *Shāng Hán Lùn,* where it is given as a treatment for *huò luàn* 霍亂 (i.e., simultaneous vomiting and diarrhea, of which cholera is a specific type.), by treating vacuity cold in the spleen and stomach with center-warming, qì-boosting, cold-dispelling medicinals.

大黄湯《千金要方衍義》

（一）方下所治少小風癇，明是木邪內盛，乘克中土。殊非外風襲入之謂。

（二）故於理中方內除去白朮之滯、甘草之緩，但取參、薑，參入細辛以散內盛之風。

（三）當歸以調紊亂之血，甘皮以豁壅遏之痰，大黄以滌固結之積。

（四）與黄龍湯同一手筆。彼以病氣盤錯，胃氣傷殘，雖用硝黄徒增脹滿，必藉人參大力，以鼓盪練之威。

（五）此以孩提血氣未實，不勝病氣留逮，雖宜大黄迅掃，必兼參、薑溫散，可無傷中之虞。

（六）然此僅堪為智者道，難使庸俗知也。

Dàhuáng Tāng (Rhubarb Decoction) *Yǎn Yì* (Expanded Meaning), cont.

(4) This formula comes from the same brush as[2] Huáng Lóng Tāng.[3] That formula takes the complex nature of the disease qì and the damage already done to stomach qì as the reason why it must rely on the great strength of *rénshēn* to drum up the might of its sweeping and thrashing action, even though the use of *mángxiāo* and *dàhuáng* uselessly increases the swelling and fullness.

(5) Regarding the present formula, it takes the fact that blood and qì are not yet replete in infants and that they are unable to overcome the lingering aspects and speedy actions of the disease qì[4] as the reason why even though the swift sweeping effect of *dàhuáng* is appropriate, it must be combined with the warm dispersing action of *rénshēn* and *gānjiāng*, so that you do not have to worry about damaging the center.

(6) Thus this formula is something that can only serve as the Way for those with wisdom, but is difficult to comprehend for more vulgar minds.

---

2 I.e., is closely related to.

3 The identity of Huáng Lóng Tāng 黄龍湯 (literally, "Yellow Dragon Decoction") here is somewhat obscure. While a medicinal formula with this name from early medieval times does exist, namely a formula mentioned by Táo Hóngjǐng in his *Zhǒu Hòu Fāng* 《肘後方》("Prescriptions to Carry Up One's Sleeve"), it consists of nothing but feces, stored in a clay container for many months until well fermented. The resulting juice is said to eliminate all toxins. Given the lack of other ingredients, this is an unlikely candidate for this reference. A more likely choice is the formula for Huáng Lóng Tāng found in a Míng period text called *Shāng Hán Liù Shū* 《傷寒六書》("Six Writings on Cold Damage") by Táo Huá 陶華. Used for hardness and pain below the heart, clear-fluid diarrhea (or constipation), delirious speech, thirst, and generalized heat that are related to dryness in center earth, the formula contains *dàhuáng*, *mángxiāo*, *zhǐshí*, *hòupò*, *gāncǎo*, *rénshēn*, and *dāngguī* and is indicated for heat binding in Yángmíng with insufficiency of qì and blood. It is an example of the treatment strategy of simultaneous attack and supplementation (*gōng bǔ jiān shī* 攻补兼施).

4 *Liú sù* 留速: The problem is a combination of stagnation and the resultant wind that arises from its transformation.

白羊鮮湯

治小兒風癇，胸中有痰方。

白羊鮮	三銖
蚱蟬	二枚
大黃	四銖
甘草	二銖
鉤藤皮	二銖
細辛	二銖
牛黃	如大豆四枚
蛇蛻	皮一寸

上八味，㕮咀，以水二升半，煮取一升二合。分五服，日三。若服已盡而癇不斷者，可更加大黃、鉤藤各一銖，以水漬藥半日，然後煮之。

III.6 Báiyángxiān Tāng (Dictamnus Decoction)

Indications

A formula for small children, to treat wind seizures with racing[1] in the center of the chest.

Ingredients

báiyángxiān	3 *zhū*
zhàchán	2 pcs
dàhuáng	4 *zhū*
gāncǎo	2 *zhū*
gōuténgpí	2 *zhū*
xìxīn	2 *zhū*
niúhuáng	4 pcs about the size of soybeans
shétuì	1 *cùn* of the skin

Preparation

Pound the eight ingredients above and decoct in 2.5 *shēng* of water until reduced to 1 *shēng* and 2 *gě*. Divide into five doses and take three times a day. If you have finished up all the doses and yet the seizures have not stopped, you can add an additional 1 *zhū* each of *dàhuáng* and *gōuténg*, soaking the medicinals in water for half a day and decocting them afterwards.

1 *Jí* 疾 can mean either "racing" (as in *jí mài* 疾脈, a racing pulse) or simply "disease" or "hardship." In that case, the entire phrase could be interpreted more generally as "with hardship in the center of the chest."

白羊鮮湯《千金要方衍義》

（一）白羊鮮即白鮮皮。《本經》雖主頭風黃癉濕痺死肌，乃兼搜風濕痰氣之藥，不獨治外證也。

（二）蚱蟬、蛇蛻、牛黃，《本經》皆主驚癇癲病。細辛疏利九竅，大黃推陳致新，甘草解毒除邪。

（三）以風癇為足厥陰之病，故用鈎藤為響導也。

Báiyángxiān Tāng (Dictamnus Decoction) *Yǎn Yì* (Expanded Meaning)

(1) *Báiyángxiān* is identical to *báixiānpí*. Although the *Shén Nóng Běn Cǎo Jīng* [describes it as] governing head wind, jaundice, damp impediment, and dead flesh, it also simultaneously serves as a medicinal that tracks down wind, dampness, and phlegm qì, and it doesn't only treat external patterns.

(2) In the *Shén Nóng Běn Cǎo Jīng*, *zhàchán*, *shétuì*, and *niúhuáng* are all indicated for fright seizures and *diān* insanity. *Xìxīn* disinhibits the nine orifices, *dàhuáng* pushes out the old to welcome the new, and *gāncǎo* resolves toxins and eliminates evil.

(3) [Lastly,] since wind seizures are a foot Juéyīn disease, we use *gōuténg* as guide.

增損續命湯

治小兒卒中風惡毒及久風，四肢角弓反張不隨，並軃曳僻，不能行步方。

麻黃	一兩
甘草	一兩
桂心	一兩
芎藭	十八銖
葛根	十八銖
升麻	十八銖
當歸	十八銖
獨活	十八銖
人參	半兩
黃芩	半兩
石膏	半兩
杏仁	二十枚

（一）上十二味，㕮咀，以水六升煮麻黃，去上沫，乃納諸藥，煮取一升二合。

（二）三歲兒分為四服，一日令盡。

（三）少取汗，得汗，以粉粉之。

III.7 Zēng Sǔn Xù Mìng Tāng (Modified Life-Prolonging Decoction)

Indications

A formula for small children, to treat sudden wind strike, malignity poisoning, and chronic wind, with arched-back rigidity and paralysis in the four limbs, as well as drooping, dragging, or deviation, and inability to walk.

Ingredients

máhuáng	1 *liǎng*
gāncǎo	1 *liǎng*
guìxīn	1 *liǎng*
xiōngqióng	18 *zhū*
gégēn	18 *zhū*
shēngmá	18 *zhū*
dāngguī	18 *zhū*
dúhuó	18 *zhū*
rénshēn	0.5 *liǎng*
huángqín	0.5 *liǎng*
shígāo	0.5 *liǎng*
xìngrén	20 pcs

Preparation

(1) Pound the twelve ingredients above. Decoct the *máhuáng* in 6 *shēng* of water, remove the foam from the top, add all the other ingredients, and decoct again until reduced to 1 *shēng* and 2 *gě*.

(2) For a child of three *suì*, divide it into four doses, and use it all up in a single day.

(3) Induce slight sweating, and once you have obtained sweating, sprinkle rice flour on the child.

增損續命湯《千金要方衍義》

（一）小兒卒中風惡毒角弓反張，皆腠理疏豁致病，故於續命。

（二）本方，增入升麻、獨活，佐麻黃以祛賊風，黃芩佐石膏以解風熱。

（三）小兒本無內虛，故損去乾薑之辛烈，不使真陰受困耳。

Zēng Sŭn Xù Mìng Tāng (Modified Life-Prolonging Decoction) *Yăn Yì* (Expanded Meaning)

(1) In small children, sudden wind strike, malignity poisoning, and arched-back rigidity are all due to the interstices being loose and gaping, which causes these diseases, hence [the present formula is based on the] Xù Mìng Tāng [formula family].[1]

(2) To the original formula, we add *shēngmá* and *dúhuó* to assist *máhuáng* in dispelling bandit wind, and *huángqín* to assist *shígāo* in resolving the wind heat.

(3) Small children originally do not suffer from internal vacuity, and we therefore remove the acrid fierceness of *gānjiāng*, to prevent encumbering true yīn.

1 For more information and modifications of formulas in the Xù Mìng Tāng family, see *Qiān Jīn Fāng* volume 8, chapter 2 on "The Various Winds."

石膏湯

治小兒中風惡疿，不能語，口眼了戾，四肢不隨方。

石膏	一合
麻黄	八銖
甘草	四銖
射乾	四銖
桂心	四銖
芍藥	四銖
當歸	四銖
細辛	二銖

（一）上八味，㕮咀，以水三升半，先煮麻黄三沸，去上沫，納餘藥，煮取一升。

（二）三歲兒分四服，日三。

III.8 Shígāo Tāng (Gypsum Decoction)

Indications

A formula for small children, to treat wind strike with malign *féi* disablement,[1] inability to speak, twisted mouth and eyes, and paralysis in the four limbs.

Ingredients

shígāo	1 *gě*
máhuáng	8 *zhū*
gāncǎo	4 *zhū*
shègān	4 *zhū*
guìxīn	4 *zhū*
sháoyào	4 *zhū*
dāngguī	4 *zhū*
xìxīn	2 *zhū*

Preparation

(1) Pound the eight ingredients above. First decoct the *máhuáng* in 3.5 *shēng* of water, bringing it to a boil three times. Remove the foam from the top, add the other medicinals, and decoct until reduced to 1 *shēng*.

(2) For a child of three *suì*, divide [the decoction] into four doses and take three doses per day.

---

1 This is the name of a condition that is the after-effect of wind strike, resembling hemilateral withering. In addition to the symptoms listed above, it can manifest with clouded consciousness. According to *Líng Shū* 《靈樞》 ("Divine Pivot," one of the two major parts of the *Huáng Dì Neì Jīng*), chapter 23 on Heat Disease, "*Féi* disablement is a disease that manifests with no pain in the body but loss of use in the four limbs. If the mental confusion is not too great and the patient's speech is still somewhat coherent, it is treatable. If the condition is severe and the patient is unable to speak, it is untreatable. The disease first arises in yáng and then enters yīn..."

石膏湯《千金要方衍義》

（一）此即排風湯之變方，於中裁去川芎、杏仁、茯苓、白朮、防風、獨活、白鮮、生薑，加入石膏、細辛、射乾。

（二）較排風湯頭緒頗清，然排風本諸續命，原有石膏。

（三）以小兒本非虛寒致病，人參、乾薑似可無藉，但石膏湯中射乾當必因腹中邪逆，或兼喉痺咽痛而設。

（四）若無上証，何復用此寒降之品也。

Shígāo Tāng (Gypsum Decoction) *Yǎn Yì* (Expanded Meaning)

(1) This formula is in fact a variation of Pái Fēng Tāng,[1] with *chuānxiōng, xìngrén, fúlíng, báizhú, fángfēng, dúhuó, báixiān*, and *shēngjiāng* removed from it and *shígāo, xìxīn,* and *shègān* added.

(2) In comparison with Pái Fēng Tāng, the main thread [of the present formula] is rather clear. Nevertheless, Pái Fēng Tāng is rooted in the various Xù Mìng Tāng [formulas], which originally contain *shígāo*.

(3) Since small children at the root do not have the problem of vacuity cold causing disease, we apparently do not have to rely on *rénshēn* and *gānjiāng*, but the *shègān* in Shígāo Tāng is indispensable because of the evil counterflow in the abdomen, which is possibly complicated by throat impediment causing throat pain.

(4) If the patient does not have the above pattern, what use would there be for this cold down-bearing substance?

1 Pái Fēng Tāng 排風湯 (Wind-Eliminating Decoction): The earliest received source for this formula is most likely the *Qiān Jīn Fāng* in vol. 8, chapter 2 on "The Various Winds." The formula includes the following ingredients: *báixiānpí, baízhú, sháoyào, guìxīn, xiōngqióng, dāngguī, xìngrén, fángfēng, gāncǎo* (2 *liǎng* each), *dúhuó, máhuáng, fúlíng* (3 *liǎng* each), and *shēngjiāng* (4 *liǎng*). See that chapter for the long list of indications for this formula, as well as for a number of related formulas to be used in similar conditions.

治少小中風，狀如欲絕湯方。

大黃	十二銖
牡蠣	十二銖
龍骨	十二銖
栝蔞根	十二銖
甘草	十二銖
桂心	十二銖
赤石脂	六銖
寒水石	六銖

（一）上八味，㕮咀，以水一升，納藥重半兩，煮再沸，絞去滓。

（二）半歲兒服如雞子大一枚，大兒盡服，入口中即愈。汗出粉之。藥無毒，可服日二。

（三）有熱加大黃，不汗加麻黃。無寒水石，朴硝代之。

III.9 Unnamed Formula

Indication

A decoction formula that treats wind strike in early childhood, with an appearance as if the patient were on the verge of expiry.

Ingredients

dàhuáng	12 *zhū*
mǔlì	12 *zhū*
lónggǔ	12 *zhū*
guālóugēn	12 *zhū*
gāncǎo	12 *zhū*
guìxīn	12 *zhū*
chìshízhī	6 *zhū*
hánshuǐshí	6 *zhū*

Preparation

(1) Pound the eight ingredients above. Using 1 *shēng* of water, add 0.5 *liǎng* in weight of the medicinals and decoct them, letting them come to a boil twice. Wring out and remove the dregs.

(2) For a six-month-old child, give an amount the size of a chicken egg per dose; for an older child, give the entire preparation as a dose. The patient will recover as soon as the medicine enters the mouth. Upon sweating, dust the patient with [rice] flour. This medicine is non-toxic and can be taken twice in a single day.

(3) For patients with heat, add *dàhuáng*; for patients who fail to sweat, add *máhuáng*. If you do not have *hánshuǐshí*, you can use *pòxiāo* as a substitute.

《千金要方衍義》

（一）此即風引湯之變方。《金匱》本治大人風引，小兒驚癇立方命名。

（二）專在引風內洩，故用大黃、甘草、寒水石。杜風復入，故用龍骨、牡蠣、赤石脂。

（三）《千金》取治小兒中風，雖風虛燥熱狀如欲絕，然不致擾亂血脈。故於本方除去四石，僅留赤石脂、寒水石，以杜風潤燥，並進栝蔞根而進乾薑。

（四）單取桂心一味，為反諜其間，淺深權度，可默識矣。

Unnamed Formula *Yǎn Yì* (Expanded Meaning)

(1) This formula is in fact a variation of Fēng Yǐn Tāng.[1] The *Jīn Guì Yào Lüè* originally established this formula and named it as such as a treatment for drawing wind in adults and for fright seizures in small children.

(2) [That original formula] is aimed specifically at drawing wind and draining it internally. Therefore it uses *dàhuáng, gāncǎo,* and *hánshuǐshí*. To block wind from entering again, it uses *lónggǔ, mǔlì,* and *chìshízhī*.

(3) Regarding its use in the *Qiān Jīn Fāng* to treat wind strike in small children, even though the wind vacuity and dry heat look like imminent expiry, the condition has not yet led to disorderly flow in the blood vessels. Therefore the present formula has eliminated four mineral substances, only leaving *chìshízhī* and *hánshuǐshí*, to shut out wind and moisten dryness. At the same time, *guālóugēn* is added and *gānjiāng* removed.[2]

(4) [The formula] uses *guìxīn* as a single ingredient to act as a spy in their midst, gauging the depth or shallowness [of the invading wind], which can be secretly known by this!

---

1 Fēng Yǐn Tāng 風引湯 ("Wind-Drawing Decoction") is a group of formulas that are presented in the *Qiān Jīn Fāng* in vol. 7 ("Wind Toxin Foot Qì"), chapter 2 ("On Decoctions and Fluids"). The actual formula called Fēng Yǐn Tāng as such is indicated for "pain, impediment, and swelling in both legs, possibly numbness, hypertonicity, and bending causing inability to walk." It contains the following ingredients: *máhuáng, shígāo, dúhuó, fúlíng* (2 *liǎng* each), *wúzhūyú, qīnjiāo, xìxīn, guìxīn, rénshēn, fángfēng, xiōngqióng, fángjǐ, gāncǎo* (1 *liǎng* each), *gānjiāng* (1.5 *liǎng*), *báizhú* (3 *liǎng*), *xìngrén* (60 pcs), *fùzǐ* (1 *liǎng*). This formula differs substantially from the older and probably more well-known one with the same name that is originally quoted in the *Jīn Guì Yào Lüè* ("Essentials from the Golden Cabinet"), an important formula collection compiled by Zhāng Zhòngjǐng in the Hàn period. That formula is intended to clear heat, extinguish wind, settle fright, and calm the spirit.

2 *Jìn gān jiāng* 進乾薑 means translated literally "*gānjiāng* added." This makes no sense in the present context since the formula in the *Qiān Jīn Fāng* does not contain *gānjiāng*. Given the suspicious grammatical construction of this sentence here and the fact that the version of Fēng Yǐn Tāng in the *Qiān Jīn Fāng* in volume 7 does in fact contain *gānjiāng*, this must be a textual error in the current edition of the *Qiān Jīn Fāng Yǎn Yì*, and *jìn* 進 ("added") should most likely be read as *qù* 去 ("removed"). I have translated accordingly.

二物石膏湯

治少小中風，手足拘急方。

石膏	如雞子大一枚，碎
真珠	一兩

上以水二升，煮石膏五六沸，納真珠，煮取一升，稍稍分服之。

衍義

（一）少小中風手足拘急，乃驚癇瘛瘲漸次。

（二）然必別有心胸熱邪証現。

（三）故專取石膏以化胸中之熱，真珠以清心包之邪，不使留泊，而為將來之變端也。

III.10 Èr Wù Shígāo Tāng (Two Ingredients Gypsum Decoction)

Indication

A formula that treats wind strike in early childhood with hypertonicity in the hands and feet.

Ingredients

shígāo	a piece the size of a chicken egg, broken into pieces
zhēnzhū	1 *liǎng*

Preparation

Of the ingredients above, decoct the *shígāo* in 2 *shēng* of water, bringing it to a boil five or six times. Add the *zhēnzhū* and decoct until reduced to 1 *shēng*. Take it in separate doses, sipping a little at a time.

Yǎn Yì (Expanded Meaning)

(1) Wind strike with hypertonicity in the hands and feet in early childhood is really a condition that gradually develops into fright seizures with tugging and slackening.

(2) Nevertheless, you must in addition also see manifestations of the pattern of heat evil in the heart and chest.

(3) For this reason, the formula specifically uses *shígāo* to transform the heat in the chest, and *zhēnzhū* to clear the evil in the pericardium. [In this way,] it prevents [these pathogens] from mooring here and becoming a disturbance in the future.

桂枝湯

治少小中風，脈浮發熱，自汗出，項強，鼻鳴乾嘔方。

桂心	一兩
甘草	一兩
芍藥	一兩
大棗	四枚
生薑	一兩

上五味，㕮咀三物，以水三升，煮取一升，分三服。

III.11 Guìzhī Tāng (Cinnamon Twig Decoction)

Indications

A formula that treats wind strike in early childhood, with a floating pulse, heat effusion, spontaneous sweating, rigidity in the neck, sounds in the nose, and dry retching.

Ingredients[1]

guìxīn	1 *liǎng*
gāncǎo	1 *liǎng*
sháoyào	1 *liǎng*
dàzǎo	4 pcs
shēngjiāng	1 *liǎng*

Preparation

Of the five ingredients above, pound the first three ingredients. Decoct [all ingredients] in 3 *shēng* of water until reduced to 1 *shēng* and divide into 3 doses.[2]

1 Contrary to the version in all other received texts and also the original source in the *Shāng Hán Lùn*《傷寒論》("Treatise on Cold Damage"), the *Sūn Zhēn Rén* edition calls for 1 *fēn* of *dàhuáng* here instead of 1 *liǎng* of *shēngjiāng*.)

2 This formula is repeated in volume 9 on "Cold Damage," chapter 5 on "Decoctions that Promote Sweating."

二物驢毛散

治少小新生中風方。

驢毛	一把，取背前交脊上會中，拔取如手拇指大一把
麝香	二豆大

（一）上以乳汁和，銅器中微火煎令焦熟出，為末。

（二）小兒不能飲，以乳汁和之，葦筒貯，瀉著咽中，然後飲乳，令入腹。

《千金要方衍義》

（一）驢肉動風，而驢毛反能治風，風氣皆發於毛。

（二）猶麋肉痿陽，而麋角力能助陽，陽精鍾聚於角也。

（三）加以麝臍通達經脈，外內無所不透，總取血肉之性，不傷初生之氣也。

III.12 Èr Wù Lümáo Săn (Two Ingredient Donkey Hair Powder)

Indications

A formula that treats wind strike in early childhood and right after birth.

Ingredients

lümáo	handful, taken from the anterior back where the mane meets the spine, pull out a thumbsized handful
shèxiāng	a piece the size of two beans

Preparation

(1) Mix the above ingredients into breast milk and brew in a copper vessel over a small flame until [the mixture] is scorched. When it is done, remove it [from the pot] and pulverize it.

(2) For small children who are unable to drink, mix it into breast milk, draw it up into a tube made out of reed, and then pour it down [the baby's] throat. Afterwards have the baby drink breast milk to make the medicine enter the belly.

Yăn Yì (Expanded Meaning)

(1) Donkey meat stirs up wind, but donkey hair is on the contrary able to treat wind, [since] all wind qì effuses through the hair.

(2) We can compare this to the way in which *míròu*[1] wilts yáng, while *míjiăo* has the force to assist yáng. The reason for this is that yáng essence is concentrated in the horn.

(3) Add to this the freeing and out-thrusting effect of *shèxiāng*[2] on the channels, and there is no place left on the outside or inside of the body that is not penetrated and no place that does not absorb the inherent nature of flesh and blood, without, however, damaging the newborn's qì.

---

1 *Míròu* 麋肉 refers to the meat of elaphure, a species of tailed deer only found in China. *Míjiăo* 麋角 ("elaphure horn") similarly refers to the horn of the same species.

2 *Shèqí*, as this substance is referred to in the *Yăn Yì* text, literally refers to the "navel of the musk deer." As a description of the location of the scent gland, this is simply an alternate way of referring to *shèxiāng* (musk).

茵芋丸

治少小有風癇疾，至長不除，或遇天陰節變便發動，食飲堅強亦發，百脈攣縮，行步不正，言語不便者，服之永不發方。

茵芋葉	一兩
鉛丹	一兩
秦艽	一兩
鈎藤皮	一兩
石膏	一兩
杜蘅	一兩
防葵	一兩
菖蒲	一兩半
黄芩	一兩半
松蘿	半兩
蜣螂	十枚
甘草	二兩

（一）上十二味，末之，蜜丸如小豆大。

（二）三歲以下服五丸，三歲以上服七丸，五歲以上服十丸，十歲以上可至十五丸。

III.13 Yīnyù Wán (Skimmia Pill)

Indications

A formula to treat [patients who suffered from] wind seizures in early childhood and have reached adulthood without getting rid of them, with outbreaks possibly triggered by gloomy weather or seasonal changes, or also by a firm and solid diet,[1] contractions in the hundred vessels, inability to walk straight, and impeded speech. After taking this formula, the disease will never break out again.

Ingredients

yīnyùyè	1 *liǎng*
qiāndān	1 *liǎng*
qínjiāo	1 *liǎng*
gōuténgpí	1 *liǎng*
shígāo	1 *liǎng*
dùhéng	1 *liǎng*
fángkuí	1 *liǎng*
chāngpú	1.5 *liǎng*
huángqín	1.5 *liǎng*
sōngluó	0.5 *liǎng*
qiāngláng	10 pcs
gāncǎo	2 *liǎng*

Preparation

(1) Pulverize the twelve ingredients above and make honey pills the size of aduki beans.

(2) For children under the age of 3 *suì*, a dose is five pills; for children above the age of 3 *suì*, a dose is 7 pills; for children above the age of 5 *suì*, a dose is 10 pills; for children above the age of 10 *suì*, you may give up to 15 pills [per dose].

1 I.e., hard-to-digest substances, like cold and raw foods.

茵芋丸《千金要方衍義》

（一）風癇而至長不出，以成固疾，非峻搜病根，何以求其克應？然須元氣稍堪勝任毒藥者，庶可圖治。

（二）茵芋為風癇專藥，《本經》治五臟心腹寒熱，然世罕識此頗不易得。

（三）鉛丹為鎮驚專藥，《本經》治驚癇癲疾，取其鎮墜頑痰也。

（四）秦艽為治風逐濕專藥，《本經》治熱邪氣、寒濕風痺，取其能散風毒也。

（五）鈎藤為小兒驚癇專藥，雖無《本經》可考，以意逆之，取其專走厥陰，風癇乃厥陰之病也。

（六）石膏為清利風熱專藥，《本經》治中風寒熱心下逆氣，驚喘，取其能除胃熱也。

（七）杜蘅為杜風祛熱專藥，《本經》治胸膈下逆氣，取其能溫中也。

（八）防葵為流走經脈專藥，《本經》治癲癇，風邪狂走，取其善通結滯也。

Yīnyù Wán (Skimmia Pill) *Yǎn Yì* (Expanded Meaning)

(1) Wind seizures that do not exit the body even upon reaching adulthood have thereby become a chronic condition. How could you therefore not fiercely search for the root of the disease in order to pursue a response to conquer it? Nevertheless, the *yuán qì* ("original qì") must be able to endure toxic medicines that are capable of succeeding at this task so that we can attempt treatment.

(2) *Yīnyù* is a medicinal used specifically for wind seizures and, according to the *Shén Nóng Běn Cǎo Jīng,* treats cold and heat in the five *zàng* organs, heart, and abdomen. Nevertheless, this is rarely known in this world and it is not easy to come by.

(3) *Qiāndān* is a medicinal used specifically for settling fright and, according to the *Shén Nóng Běn Cǎo Jīng,* treats fright seizures and *diān* insanity disease. It is chosen [here] for its ability to settle and press down obstinate phlegm.

(4) *Qínjiāo* is a medicinal used specifically for treating wind and expelling dampness and, according to the *Shén Nóng Běn Cǎo Jīng,* treats the evil qì of heat, and cold, damp, and wind impediment. It is chosen [here] for its ability to disperse wind toxin.

(5) *Gōuténg* is a medicinal used specifically for fright seizures in small children. Even though it cannot be researched in the *Shén Nóng Běn Cǎo Jīng,* we can predict [its effect] with our mind. It is chosen [here] because it specifically moves through Juéyīn, and wind seizures are a Juéyīn disease.

(6) *Shígāo* is a medicinal used specifically for clearing and disinhibiting wind heat and, according to the *Shén Nóng Běn Cǎo Jīng,* treats wind strike with cold and heat, counterflow qì below the heart, and fright panting. It is chosen [here] because of its ability to eliminate heat from the stomach.

(7) *Dùhéng* is a medicinal used specifically for shutting out wind and driving out heat. According to the *Shén Nóng Běn Cǎo Jīng,* it treats counterflow qì below the chest and diaphragm. It is selected [here] for its ability to warm the center.

茵芋丸《千金要方衍義》

（七）杜蘅為杜風祛熱專藥，《本經》治胸膈下逆氣，取其能溫中也。

（八）防葵為流走經脈專藥，《本經》治癲癇，風邪狂走，取其善通結滯也。

（九）菖蒲為開通心氣專藥，《本經》治風寒溫痺，取其能利九竅也。

（十）黃芩為分解風熱專藥，《本經》治逐水下血閉，取其專行少陽也。

（十一）松蘿為鬆上女蘿，為去風平肝專藥，《本經》治癲怒邪氣，取且善療風熱也。

（十二）蜣蜋為撥毒散結專藥，《本經》治小兒驚癇瘈瘲，大人癲疾狂陽，取其力破痰血也。

（十三）甘草為和中解毒專藥，《本經》治五臟六腑寒熱邪氣，取其調和諸藥也。

（十四）合諸性味參之，則永不復發之功，可想望矣。

Yīnyù Wán (Skimmia Pill) *Yǎn Yì* (Expanded Meaning), cont.

(8) *Fángkuí* is a medicinal used specifically for promoting movement and flow in the channels and, according to the *Shén Nóng Běn Cǎo Jīng*, treats *diān* insanity and seizures, and manically running wind evil with manic running. It is selected [here] for its skill in opening up binds and stagnations.

(9) *Chāngpú* is a medicinal used specifically for opening up heart qì and, according to the *Shén Nóng Běn Cǎo Jīng*, treats wind, cold, and warmth impediment. It is selected here for its ability to disinhibit the nine orifices.

(10) *Huángqín* is a medicinal used specifically for separating and resolving wind and heat. According to the *Shén Nóng Běn Cǎo Jīng*, it cures by expelling water and moving blood blockages downward. It is selected [here] for its ability to specifically go into Shàoyáng.

(11) *Sōngluó* is the lichen growing on pine trees and a medicinal used specifically for getting rid of wind and balancing the liver. According to the *Shén Nóng Běn Cǎo Jīng*, it treats the evil qì of *diān* insanity and rage. It is selected [here] moreover for its ability to cure wind heat.

(12) *Qiāngláng* is a medicinal used specifically for stirring up toxins and dispersing binds. According to the *Shén Nóng Běn Cǎo Jīng*, it treats fright seizures with tugging and slackening in small children, and *diān* insanity disease with manic yáng in adults. It is selected [here] for its force in breaking up phlegm and blood.

(13) *Gāncǎo* is a medicinal used specifically for harmonizing the center and resolving toxins. According to the *Shén Nóng Běn Cǎo Jīng*, it treats evil qì of cold and heat in the five *zàng* and six *fǔ* organs. It is selected [here] for its ability to harmonize all the other ingredients.

(14) When we combine all these ingredients with their special characteristics to work together, they have the effect of never allowing another relapse. This is what we hope for!

鎮心丸

治小兒驚癎百病，鎮心氣方。

銀屑	十二銖
水銀	二十銖
牛黄	六銖
大黄	六分
茯苓	三分
茯神	二分
遠志	二分
防己	二分
白蘞	二分
雄黄	二分
人參	二分
芍藥	二分
防葵	四分
鐵精	四分
紫石英	四分
真珠	四分

（一）上十六味，先以水銀和銀屑如泥，別治諸藥，和丸。三歲兒如麻子二丸，隨兒大小增之。

III.14 Zhèn Xīn Wán (Heart-Settling Pill)

Indication

A formula for small children to treat the hundred diseases of fright seizures by settling heart qì.

Ingredients

yínxiè	12 *zhū*
shuǐyín	20 *zhū*
niúhuáng	6 *zhū*
dàhuáng	6 *fēn*
fúlíng	3 *fēn*
fúshén	2 *fēn*
yuǎnzhì	2 *fēn*
fángjǐ	2 *fēn*
báiliǎn	2 *fēn*
xiónghuáng	2 *fēn*
rénshēn	2 *fēn*
sháoyào	2 *fēn*
fángkuí	4 *fēn*
tiějīng	4 *fēn*
zǐshíyīng	4 *fēn*
zhēnzhū	4 *fēn*

Preparation

(1) Of the sixteen ingredients above, first combine the *shuǐyín* and *yínxiè* [and process them] into a mud-like consistency. Separately pestle all the other ingredients, and combine [everything] into pills. For a child of 3 *suì*, give two pills the size of hemp seeds. Increase this dosage in accordance with the child's age.[1]

1 An editorial note in some editions, presumably by the Sòng editors of the *Qiān Jīn Fāng*, states that other versions of this formula do not contain the ingredient *niúhuáng*.

鎮心丸《千金要方衍義》

（一）鎮心，而用銀屑、水銀、鐵精、雄黃、石英、真珠以鎮其怯，大黃、牛黃以滌其痰，茯苓、茯神以安其神，防己、防葵以破其結，芍藥、白蘞以收其散，人參、遠志以發其竅。

（二）竅隧利而神識清，何慮驚痰之不渙散乎？

Zhèn Xīn Wán (Heart-Settling Pill) ***Yǎn Yì*** **(Expanded Meaning)**

(1) To settle the heart, [the formula] uses *yínxiè, shuǐyín, tiějīng, xiónghuáng, zǐshíyīng,* and *zhēnzhū* to settle its timidity; *dàhuáng* and *niúhuáng* to flush out its phlegm; *fúlíng* and *fúshén* to calm its spirit; *fángjǐ* and *fángkuí* to break up its binds; *sháoyào* and *báiliǎn* to gather in its scattering; and *rénshēn* and *yuǎnzhì* to effuse its orifices.

(2) Once the orifices are tunneled free and the spirit consciousness is clear, why would you worry about fright and phlegm failing to disperse?

丹參赤膏

治少小心腹熱，除熱方。

丹參	二兩
雷丸	二兩
芒硝	二兩
戎鹽	二兩
大黃	二兩

上五味，㕮咀，以苦酒半升，浸四種一宿，以成煉豬肪一斤，煎三上三下，去滓，乃納芒硝。膏成，以摩心下，冬夏可用。

III.15 Dānshēn Chì Gāo (Red Salvia Salve)

Indications

A formula that treats heat in the heart and abdomen in early childhood, by eliminating the heat.

Ingredients

dānshēn	2 *liǎng*
léiwán	2 *liǎng*
mángxiāo	2 *liǎng*
róngyán	2 *liǎng*
dàhuáng	2 *liǎng*

Preparation

Pound the five ingredients above. Soak four of them[1] in 0.5 *shēng* of bitter wine[2] for one night and then heat them slowly in 1 *jīn* of rendered lard, simmering it and then taking it off the flame three times. Discard the dregs. Now add the *mángxiāo*. When the salve is done, massage it into the area below the heart. You can use it both in the winter and summer.[3]

---

1 I.e., everything but the *mángxiāo*, which is added later in the process.

2 *Kǔ jiǔ* 苦酒: I purposely translate this phrase literally here as "bitter wine," even though it is commonly used and interpreted in later formulary literature as a gloss for *cù* 醋 ("vinegar"). In classical times, this was not necessarily the case and the term referred to a different substance, most likely simply wine that had gone bad. The chapter on "Explaining Food and Drinks" in the *Shì Míng*《释名》("Explaining Names," a text from the end of the Hàn period) explains: "Bitter wine: A substance with a great concentration of toxicity (i.e., alcohol), both vinegary and bitter" "苦酒：淳毒甚者，酢〔且〕苦也。"

3 An editorial note to the text, presumably from the Sòng period editors, adds that some versions of this formula use only *dānshēn* and *léiwán* and that this is also an excellent treatment.

丹參赤膏《千金要方衍義》

（一）小兒心腹常熱，皆母腹中瘀垢未清，血氣不和所致。

（二）故用丹參、雷丸、硝黃、戎鹽散血逐熱之藥。

（三）製為赤膏，常摩心下，使瘀散血和，其熱自除。

（四）漬用苦酒，專取峻收，以固腠理；煎用豬肪，專取脂澤，以潤肌膚也。

Dānshēn Chì Gāo (Red Salvia Salve) *Yǎn Yì* (Expanded Meaning)

(1) In small children, constant heat in the heart and abdomen is always caused by stagnant filth inside the mother's abdomen that was not cleared away and caused disharmony of blood and qì.

(2) Therefore *dānshēn, léiwán, mángxiāo, dàhuáng,* and *róngyán* are used for their medicinal effect of dispersing the blood and expelling heat.

(3) Processed into a red salve and constantly massaged into the area below the heart, [this treatment] causes the stasis to dissipate and the blood to become harmonious, as a result of which the heat is eliminated on its own.

(4) Using bitter liquor to soak the ingredients in takes advantage specifically of its fierce contracting action, in order to secure the interstices. Heating [the medicinals] slowly in lard takes advantage specifically of its fatty and lustrous nature, to moisten the skin.

五物甘草生摩膏

治少小新生，肌膚幼弱，喜為風邪所中，身體壯熱，或中大風，手足驚掣方。

甘草	一兩
防風	一兩
白朮	二十銖
雷丸	二兩半
桔梗	二十銖

（一）上五味，㕮咀。以不中水豬肪一斤，煎為膏。以煎藥，微火上煎之，消息視稠濁，膏成去滓。

（二）取如彈丸大一枚，炙手以摩兒百過。

（三）寒者更熱，熱者更寒。

（四）小兒雖無病，早起常以膏摩囟上及手足心，甚辟風寒。

III.16 Wǔ Wù Gāncǎo Shēng Mó Gāo
(Five Substances Licorice Life-Massage Salve)

Indications

A formula for very young children and newborns with delicate skin and a tendency to be struck by wind evil, [manifesting] with vigorous heat effusion all over the body and possibly, if they have been struck by major wind, with frightful tugging in the hands and feet.

Ingredients

gāncǎo	1 *liǎng*
fángfēng	1 *liǎng*
báizhú	20 *zhū*
léiwán	2.5 *liǎng*
jiégěng	20 *zhū*

Preparation

(1) Pound the five ingredients above. Take 1 *jīn* of lard that does not contain any water and simmer it down to make a paste. Use this to simmer the medicinals, simmering them over a gentle flame, increasing or decreasing [the heat] by observing the thickness and turbidity [of the mixture]. When the salve is done, remove the dregs.

(2) Take a pellet-sized piece, "roast" your hands,[1] and use them to massage the child with a hundred strokes.

(3) Cold [conditions] will change to heat; heat [conditions] will change to cold.

(4) Even if small children do not suffer from any illness, when they get up in the morning use this salve frequently to massage it into the top of their fontanels and in the center of the hands and feet. It is great for avoiding wind and cold.

---

1 I read this as an instruction to warm your hands until they are extremely hot and then immediately perform the massage. This is my best guess for the expression *zhì shǒu* 炙手, based partly on the explanation in the paragraph from the *Qiān Jīn Fāng Yǎn Yì* quoted below.

五物甘草生摩膏《千金要方衍義》

（一）生摩膏，摩兒囟門，手足以拒風寒。

（二）僅用前方中雷丸一味，入於防風、白朮、甘草、桔梗劑中，以實皮腠肌肉。

（三）故但取豬肪熬膏，無藉苦酒之峻收也。

（四）炙手時摩，不特可以杜風，并杜驚掣之患。

（五）此与赤膏皆外治之良法耳。

Wǔ Wù Gāncǎo Shēng Mó Gāo (Five Substances Licorice Life-Massage Salve) *Yǎn Yì* (Expanded Meaning)

(1) *Shēng Mó Gāo* is massaged into the child's fontanels and hands and feet in order to resist wind and cold.

(2) It only uses the single ingredient *léiwán* from the previous formula, with the addition of *fángfēng*, *báizhú*, *gāncǎo*, and *jiégěng* to the preparation, to make the skin's interstices and the flesh replete.

(3) Therefore only pig lard is chosen [as a base] to simmer the salve, without relying on the fierce contracting effect of bitter liquor.

(4) When you massage the patient with "roasting" hands, this not only enables the treatment to shut out wind but at the same time shuts out the trouble of frightful tugging.

(5) This salve and the red salve [of the previous formula] are both excellent methods for external treatments!

灸法

論曰：

（一）小兒新生無疾，慎不可逆針灸之。

（二）如逆針灸，則忍痛動其五脈，因喜成癇。

（三）河洛關中土地多寒，兒喜病痙。

（四）其生兒三日，多逆灸以防之。

（五）又灸頰以防噤。有噤者，舌下脈急，牙車筋急。

（六）其土地寒，皆決舌下去血，灸頰以防噤也。

（七）吳蜀地溫，無此疾也。

（八）古方既傳之，今人不詳南北之殊，便按方而用之，是以多害於小兒也。

（九）所以田舍小兒，任其自然，皆得無有夭橫也。

III.17 Moxibustion Treatments

III.17.1 Essay

(1) In small children and newborns who do not suffer from any illness, beware! You must not apply preventative acupuncture or moxibustion[1] in anticipation [of future pathological developments]!

(2) If you apply preventative acupuncture or moxibustion, enduring the pain will stir the five vessels[2] and they consequently develop a tendency to form seizures.

(3) The geographical areas of the Yellow and Luò Rivers and of the central Shǎnxī plain are dominated by a cold climate. Children there have a tendency to fall ill with tetany.

(4) On the third day after birth, children there are commonly treated with preventative moxibustion in order to prevent this.

(5) In addition, people burn moxa on the cheeks to prevent clenched jaw. The condition of clenched jaw manifests with hypertonicity in the sublingual vessels and in the sinews of the jaw.

(6) [Because] the lands there are cold, they always dredge [the vessels] below the tongue, getting rid of the blood, and burn moxa on the cheeks, in order to prevent clenched jaw.

(7) In Wú and Shǔ,[3] the lands are warm and this disease does not exist.

(8) The ancient method books transmitted this [method], but modern people do not pay attention to the differences between South and North. Hence they [indiscriminately] follow the method books and apply this [method]. This is the reason for much harm to small children.

(9) For this reason, small children in peasant households where things are left to nature never suffer from perverse premature death.

---

1 According to my own interpretation of *nì* 逆 here, confirmed by a modern editorial comment in the Rén Mín Wèi Shēng edition, the character should not be read as "counterflow," its more common medical connotation, but in a different sense as *wèi zhì ér yíng zhī* 未至而迎之 "welcoming something / somebody before it has arrived." The phrase *nì zhēn jiǔ* 逆針灸 then has the sense of applying preventative acupuncture or moxibustion before any illness has arisen. It is interesting to note that the *Sūn Zhēn Rén* edition does not contain the character *zhēn* 針 "acupuncture," so the text merely says "...you must not apply moxibustion..."

2 I.e., the major vessels associated with the five viscera.

3 I.e., an area in the southeast of China, roughly coinciding with the modern-day provinces of Jiāngsū and Sìchuān.

灸法

論曰：

（一）小兒驚啼，眠中四肢掣動，變蒸未解，慎不可針灸抓之。

（二）動其百脈，仍因驚成癇也。

（三）惟陰癇噤痙，可針灸抓之。

（一）凡灸癇，當先下兒使虛，乃承虛灸之。

（二）未下有實而灸者，氣逼前後不通殺人。

（一）癇發平旦者，在足少陽；晨朝發者，在足厥陰；日中發者，在足太陽。黃昏發者，在足太陰；人定發者，在足陽明；夜半發者，在足少陰。

（二）上癇發時病所在，視其發早晚，灸其所也。

III.17 Moxibustion Treatments

III.17.2 Essay

(1) When small children [suffer from] frightful crying, tugging and moving the four extremities in their sleep, and transformations and steamings that have not yet resolved, beware! You must not apply acupuncture or moxibustion to arrest [this condition].

(2) Stirring their hundred vessels, [such treatment] will only cause [more] fright and because of this form seizures.

(3) It is only in conditions of yīn seizures[1] with clenched jaw and tetany that it is permissible to apply acupuncture and moxibustion to arrest [the disease].

III.17.3 Essay

(1) Whenever you treat seizures with moxibustion, you must first induce a downward movement and make the child vacuous. Only then, on account of that vacuity, do you treat them with moxibustion.

(2) If you apply moxibustion before you have induced a downward movement and while the patient is in a state of repletion, this will force the qì [to move] forward and backward without flowing through. This kills the person.

III.17.4 Essay

(1) Seizures that erupt at dawn are located in the Foot Shàoyáng. Seizures that erupt in the morning are located in the Foot Juéyīn. Seizures that erupt at noon are located in the Foot Tàiyáng. Seizures that erupt at dusk are located in the Foot Tàiyīn. Seizures that erupt at night after people have fallen asleep are located in the Foot Yángmíng. Seizures that erupt at midnight are located in the Foot Shàoyīn.

(2) [In accordance with] the above timing of seizures and corresponding location of the disease, observe the time of day of outbreaks and then apply moxibustion to its location.

---

1 "Yīn seizures" (*yīn xiān* 陰癎) refers to a form of seizures that is associated with yīn conditions. According to the *Yòu Kē Xīn Fǎ Yào Jué*《幼科心法要诀》("Crucial Tricks from the Heart in Pediatrics," an important Qing dynasty classic on pediatrics recorded in the *Yī Zōng Jīn Jiàn*《医宗金鉴》), "yīn seizures are associated with reversal cold in the *zàng* organs and extremities, a supine body position with hypertonicity and a white or green-blue face, vomiting foam with faint sounds, and a fine sunken pulse. It is treated by means of spleen-moving (*xíng pí* 行脾), true [qì]-securing (*gù zhēn* 固真), and seizure-settling (*dìng xiān* 定癎) preparations."

（一）癇有五臟之癇，六畜之癇，或在四肢，或在腹內。

（二）審其候，隨病所在灸之，雖少必瘥。

（三）若失其要，則為害也。

III.18 Moxibustion Treatment Of Seizures In Accordance With Differentiation By Association With *Zàng* Organs Or Domestic Animals

III.18.1 Introduction

(1) Seizures can be differentiated into seizures of the five *zàng* organs, seizures of the six domestic animals, and whether they are located in the four extremities or inside the abdomen.

(2) Examine the signs [of the seizures] and then apply moxibustion in accordance with the location of the disease. [If you follow this principle,] even though the patient may be young, he or she will invariably recover.

(3) If you lose sight of this principle, you will cause harm.

（一）肝癇之為病，面青，目反視，手足搖。灸足少陽、厥陰各三壯。

（二）心癇之為病，面赤，心下有熱，短氣，息微數。灸心下第二肋端宛宛中，此為巨闕也。又灸手心主及少陰各三壯。

（三）脾癇之為病，面黃，腹大，喜痢。灸胃脘三壯，挾胃管旁灸二壯，足陽明、太陰各二壯。

（四）肺癇之為病，面目白，口沫出。灸肺俞三壯，又灸手陽明、太陰各二壯。

（五）腎癇之為病，面黑，正直視不搖如尸狀。灸心下二寸二分三壯，又灸肘中動脈各二壯。又灸足太陽、少陰各二壯。

（六）膈癇之為病，目反，四肢不舉。灸風府，又灸頂上、鼻人中、下唇承漿，皆隨年壯。

（七）腸癇之為病，不動搖。灸兩承山，又灸足心、兩手勞宮，又灸兩耳後完骨，各隨年壯。又灸臍中五十壯。

（八）上五臟癇証候。

III.18 Moxibustion Treatment Of Seizures In Accordance With Differentiation By Association With *Zàng* Organs Or Domestic Animals

III.18.2 Differentiation by Internal Organs

(1) When the disease is liver seizures, it manifests in a green-blue face, backward-staring eyes, and shaking hands and feet. Apply moxibustion to Foot Shàoyáng and Juéyīn, three cones each.

(2) When the disease is heart seizures, it manifests in a red face, the presence of heat below the heart, shortness of breath, and faint rapid breathing. Apply moxibustion on the end of the second rib below the heart in the middle of the prominent curve. This is Jùquè ("Great Tower Gate").[1] In addition, apply moxibustion to Hand Heart-Ruler[2] and Shàoyīn, three cones each.

(3) When the disease is spleen seizures, it manifests in a yellow face, enlarged abdomen, and a tendency to diarrhea. To treat with moxibustion, burn three cones on the stomach cavity and two cones to the sides of the stomach duct.[3] Apply moxibustion also to Foot Yángmíng and Tàiyīn, two cones each.

(4) When the disease is lung seizures, it manifests in a white face and eyes and foaming from the mouth. To treat with moxibustion, burn three cones on the lung transport points and also burn two cones each on Hand Yángmíng and Tàiyīn.

(5) When the disease is kidney seizures, it manifests in a black face, directly forward-staring eyes, no shaking, and a corpse-like appearance. To treat with moxibustion, burn three cones 2 *cùn* and 2 *fēn* below the heart, and also burn two cones each on the stirring vessel in the middle of the elbow. Also, apply moxibustion to Foot Tàiyáng and Shàoyīn, two cones each.

---

1 This name is now associated with the modern point REN-14, which is described as being located on the center line of the body 6 cùn above the navel. In spite of the difference in location, the modern point is still indicated for seizures.

2 I.e., Hand Juéyīn or pericardium.

3 Rather than reading it as a literal anatomical description, *wèi wǎn* 胃脘 can also be interpreted as an alternate name for the modern point more commonly referred to as Zhōngwǎn 中脘 (Central Stomach Duct, REN-12) on the body's center line 4 *cùn* above the navel.

（一）肝癇之為病，面青，目反視，手足搖。灸足少陽、厥陰各三壯。

（二）心癇之為病，面赤，心下有熱，短氣，息微數。灸心下第二肋端宛宛中，此為巨闕也。又灸手心主及少陰各三壯。

（三）脾癇之為病，面黃，腹大，喜痢。灸胃脘三壯，挾胃管旁灸二壯，足陽明、太陰各二壯。

（四）肺癇之為病，面目白，口沫出。灸肺俞三壯，又灸手陽明、太陰各二壯。

（五）腎癇之為病，面黑，正直視不搖如尸狀。灸心下二寸二分三壯，又灸肘中動脈各二壯。又灸足太陽、少陰各二壯。

（六）膈癇之為病，目反，四肢不舉。灸風府，又灸頂上、鼻人中、下唇承漿，皆隨年壯。

（七）腸癇之為病，不動搖。灸兩承山，又灸足心、兩手勞宮，又灸兩耳後完骨，各隨年壯。又灸臍中五十壯。

（八）上五臟癇証候。

III.18 Moxibustion Treatment Of Seizures In Accordance With Differentiation By Association With *Zàng* Organs Or Domestic Animals

III.18.2 Differentiation by Internal Organs, cont.

(6) When the disease is diaphragm seizures, it manifests in backward-staring eyes and inability to lift the four extremities. Apply moxibustion to Fēngfǔ,[4] as well as to the top of the vertex, to Rénzhōng under the nose,[5] and to Chéngjiāng below the lips,[6] in each location matching the number of cones to the patient's years of age.

(7) When the disease is intestinal seizures, it manifests in the absence of moving and shaking. Apply moxibustion to the two Chéngshān points,[7] and also to the center of the feet, to the two Láogōng points on the hands,[8] and to the two Wángǔ points behind the ears,[9] in each location matching the number of cones to the patient's years of age. Also burn fifty moxa cones in the center of the navel.[10]

(8) Listed above are the signs and symptoms for seizures associated with the five *zàng* organs.

---

4 While the equation of the classical names with the modern anatomically defined points is fraught with difficulties, in cases like this, where no further information is offered regarding location, we can assume with some certainty that the point is roughly equivalent with the modern one. Fēngfǔ ("Wind Palace") is also known by its channel and associated number as DU-16. In general, the classical localization of modern acupuncture points is an issue that is in great need of more research.

5 DU-26 ("Human Center").

6 REN-24 ("Sauce Receptacle").

7 UB-57 ("Mountain Support").

8 PC-8 ("Palace of Toil").

9 GB-12 ("Completion Bone"), the mastoid processes.

10 It is not clear whether this direction refers to all cases of visceral seizures, or only to the last one. Given the large number of cones compared to the rest of the instructions, my guess is that this is a concluding sentence that should apply to all forms of visceral seizures. The modern editors of both the Rén Mín Wèi Shēng and *Huá Xià* editions disagree with me here and associate this last line with the treatment of intestinal seizures alone.

（一）馬癇之為病，張口搖頭，馬鳴，欲反折。灸項風府、臍中三壯。病在腹中，燒馬蹄末服之良。

（二）牛癇之為病，目正直視，腹脹。灸鳩尾骨及大椎各二壯。

（三）燒牛蹄末服之良。

（三）羊癇之為病，喜揚目吐舌。灸大椎上三壯。

（四）豬癇之為病，喜吐沫。灸完骨兩旁各一寸七壯。

（五）犬癇之為病，手屈拳攣。灸兩手心一壯，灸足太陽一壯，灸肋戶一壯。

（六）雞癇之為病，搖頭反折，喜驚自搖。灸足諸陽各三壯。

（七）上六畜癇証候。

III.18 Moxibustion Treatment Of Seizures In Accordance With Differentiation By Association With *Zàng* Organs Or Domestic Animals

III.18.3 Differentiation by Domestic Animal

(1) When the disease is horse seizures, it manifests in a gaping mouth and shaking head, neighing like a horse, and imminent arched-back rigidity. Apply moxibustion to Fēngfǔ on the neck and to the middle of the navel, three cones each. If the disease is located in the abdomen, ingesting pulverized charred horse hooves is excellent.

(2) When the disease is ox seizures, it manifests in directly forward-staring eyes and abdominal distention. Apply moxibustion to Jiūwěi and Dàzhuī, two cones each.[1] Ingesting pulverized charred ox hooves is excellent.

(3) When the disease is goat or sheep seizures, it manifests in a tendency to fluttering eyes and a protruding tongue. Apply moxibustion on top of Dàzhuī, three cones.

(4) When the disease is pig seizures, it manifests in a tendency to vomit foam. Apply moxibustion 1 *cùn* to both sides of Wángǔ, seven cones each.

(5) When the disease is dog seizures, it manifests in bent hands and contracted fists. Apply moxibustion to the centers of both hands, 1 cone [each]. Also apply moxibustion to Foot Tàiyáng and to Lèihù ("Rib Door"), 1 cone each.[2]

(6) When the disease is chicken seizures, it manifests in head-shaking, arched-back rigidity, a tendency to fright, and spontaneous shaking. Apply moxibustion to the various yáng [channels] on the foot, 3 cones.

(7) Listed above are the signs and symptoms for seizures associated with the six domestic animals.

---

1 REN-15 ("Turtledove Tail") and DU-14 ("Great Hammer"), respectively.

2 This is the name of a point that is no longer in common use. It is also quoted for treatment of the same condition (dog seizures in young children) in the *Zhēn Jiǔ Dà Chéng* 《針灸大成》 ("Great Compendium of Acupuncture and Moxibustion," compiled byYáng Jìzhōu 楊繼洲 and published in 1601).

（一）小兒暴癇，灸兩乳頭，女兒灸乳下二分。

（二）治小兒暴癇者，身軀正直如死人，及腹中雷鳴，灸太倉及臍中上下兩旁各一寸，凡六處。

（三）又灸當腹度取背，以繩繞頸下至臍中竭，便轉繩向背，順脊下行，盡繩頭，灸兩旁各一寸五壯。

（四）若面白，啼聲色不變，灸足陽明、太陰。

III.19 Fulminant Seizures

III.19.1

(1) For fulminant seizures in small children, apply moxibustion to both nipples. In girls, apply moxibustion 2 *fēn* below the nipples.

(2) When treating fulminant seizures in small children, [if the patient presents with] a straightened corpse-like body as well as thunderous rumbling in the abdomen, apply moxibustion to Tàicāng ("Supreme Granary") as well as 1 *cùn* each above and below and to both sides of the center of the navel, in a total of six locations.

(3) In addition, apply moxibustion to the back, using the abdomen as measurement: Take a string, wind it around the neck, and run it down to the center of the navel to mark its end. Then turn the string around to the back, follow it down along the spine, and apply moxibustion 1 *cùn* to both sides of where the string ends, five cones each.

(4) If the face is white, there is a chirping sound, and the facial complexion does not change, apply moxibustion to Foot Yángmíng and Tàiyīn.

（一）若目反上視，眸子動，當灸囟中。

（二）取之法：橫度口盡兩吻際，又橫度鼻下亦盡兩邊，折去鼻度半，都合口為度，以額上髮際上行度之，灸度頭一處，正在囟上未合骨中，隨手動者是，此最要處也。

（三）次灸當額上入髮二分許，直望鼻為正。

（四）次灸其兩邊，當目瞳子直上入髮際 二分許。

（五）次灸頂上回毛中。

（六）次灸客主人穴，在眉後際動脈是。

（七）次灸兩耳門，當耳開口則骨解開動張陷是也。

（八）次灸兩耳上，卷耳取之，當卷耳上頭是也。一法：大人當耳上橫三指，小兒各自取其指也。

（九）次灸兩耳後完骨上青脈。亦可以針刺令血出。

（十）次灸玉枕，項後高骨是也。

（十一）次灸兩風池，在項後兩轅動筋外髮際陷中是也。

（十二）次灸風府，當項中央髮際，亦可與風池三處高下相等。

（十三）次灸頭兩角，兩角當回毛兩邊起骨是也。

III.19 Fulminant Seizures

III.19.2

(1) If the eyes are turned upward and the pupils are moving, you must apply moxibustion to Xìnzhōng ("Center Fontanel").[1]

(2) Method of localizing it: Measure horizontally the full length of the mouth, from one corner of the lips to the other. Again, measure horizontally the full length below the nose [from edge to edge of] both sides [of the nostrils]. Cut the nose measurement in half. Combine this with the [length of the] mouth and take this as your measurement. Now use this to measure that same distance upward from the hairline above the forehead. Apply moxibustion to this single location on the head, which is directly on top of the fontanel in the center where the bones have not yet joined together. If you can move it with the hands, this is it. This is the most crucial location.

(3) Next, apply moxibustion to a place above the forehead, about 2 *fēn* beyond the hairline. Look straight down at the nose to place it right in the center.

(4) Next, apply moxibustion to both sides of this location: Go straight up from the pupils, about 2 *fēn* past the hairline.

(5) Next, apply moxibustion to the top of the vertex, in the center of where the hair swirls in a circle.

(6) Next, apply moxibustion to Kèzhŭrén ("Guest-Host-Person").[2] This point is located on the moving vessel at the posterior edge of the eyebrows.

(7) Next, apply moxibustion to the two Ěrmén points.[3] These points are located by the ears in the long indentation that is formed when the joint moves as the mouth is opened.

---

1 This is a point name whose description below makes it appear roughly equivalent with Xìnhuì 囟會 ("Fontanel Meeting," DU-22).

2 Presumably the modern point GB-3.

3 SJ-21 ("Ear Gate").

（一）若目反上視，眸子動，當灸囟中。

（二）取之法：橫度口盡兩吻際，又橫度鼻下亦盡兩邊，折去鼻度半，都合口為度，以額上髮際上行度之，灸度頭一處，正在囟上未合骨中，隨手動者是，此最要處也。

（三）次灸當額上入髮二分許，直望鼻為正。

（四）次灸其兩邊，當目瞳子直上入髮際 二分許。

（五）次灸頂上回毛中。

（六）次灸客主人穴，在眉後際動脈是。

（七）次灸兩耳門，當耳開口則骨解開動張陷是也。

（八）次灸兩耳上，卷耳取之，當卷耳上頭是也。一法：大人當耳上橫三指，小兒各自取其指也。

（九）次灸兩耳後完骨上青脈。亦可以針刺令血出。

（十）次灸玉枕，項後高骨是也。

（十一）次灸兩風池，在項後兩轅動筋外髮際陷中是也。

（十二）次灸風府，當項中央髮際，亦可與風池三處高下相等。

（十三）次灸頭兩角，兩角當回毛兩邊起骨是也。

III.19 Fulminant Seizures

III.19.2 cont.

(8) Next, apply moxibustion to the top of both ears. Locate the point by means of the curve of the ear, it is on the head right above the curve of the ear. Another method: In adults, go up from the ear with three fingers placed horizontally; in small children, use their own fingers.

(9) Next, apply moxibustion to the green-blue vessel above the mastoid process behind both ears. You can also use a needle to prick it until it bleeds.

(10) Next, apply moxibustion to Yùzhěn,[4] which is the elevated bone behind the nape of the neck.

(11) Next, apply moxibustion to the two Fēngchí points,[5] which are located behind the neck on the outside of the two shaft-like moving sinews, in the center of the depressions on the hairline.

(12) Next, apply moxibustion to Fēngfǔ, which is in the very center of the neck right on the hairline. You can also [locate it by] measuring equal distances to both Fēngchí points.

(13) Next, apply moxibustion to the two corners of the head. The two corners are the protruding bones on both sides where the hair swirls.

---

4 UB-9 ("Jade Pillow").
5 GB-20 ("Wind Pool").

（一）上頭部凡十九處。

（二）兒生十日可灸三壯，三十日可灸五壯，五十日可灸七壯。

（三）病重者俱灸之，輕者灸囟中、風池、玉枕也。

（四）艾使熟，炷令平正著肉，火勢乃至病所也。

（五）艾若生，炷不平正，不著肉，徒灸多炷，故無益也。

III.19 Fulminant Seizures

III.19.3

(1) Above, there are a total of nineteen locations listed for the head section.

(2) Ten days after the child's birth, you can burn three moxa cones; thirty days [after birth], you can burn five moxa cones; fifty days [after birth], you can burn seven moxa cones.

(3) If the illness is severe, burn moxa on all [of the points listed above]. If the illness is mild, burn moxa on Xìnzhōng, Fēngchí, and Yùzhěn.

(4) Make sure that the moxa is well-aged and that the cones are placed flat and directly perpendicular on the flesh so that the might of the fire indeed reaches the location of the disease.

(5) If the moxa is fresh or the cones are not placed flat and directly perpendicular on the flesh, you will burn numerous cones in vain and consequently gain no benefit at all.

（一）若腹滿短氣轉鳴，灸肺募，在兩乳上第二肋間宛宛中，懸繩取之，當瞳子是。

（二）次灸膻中。

（三）次灸胸堂。

（四）次灸臍中。

（五）次灸薜息，薜息在兩乳下，第一肋間宛宛中是也。

（六）次灸巨闕，大人去鳩尾下一寸，小兒去臍作六分分之，去鳩尾下一寸是也，並灸兩邊。

（七）次灸胃管。

（八）次灸金門，金門在穀道前，囊之後，當中央是也，從陰囊下度至大孔前，中分之。

III.19 Fulminant Seizures

III.19.4

(1) [For patients with] abdominal fullness, shortness of breath, and cramping[1] and rumbling, apply moxibustion to the lung *mù* (alarm) point. They are located above the two breasts in the space of the second rib in the middle of the curviest part. You locate it by suspending a string: Where it runs through the pupils, this is it.

(2) Next, apply moxibustion to Tánzhōng.[2]

(3) Next, apply moxibustion to Xiōngtáng ("Chest Hall").[3]

(4) Next, apply moxibustion to Qízhōng.[4]

(5) Next, apply moxibustion to Bìxī.[5] Bìxī is located below the two breasts, in the space of the first rib in the middle of the curviest part.

(6) Next, apply moxibustion to Jùquè. In adults, go down 1 *cùn* from Jiūwěi; in small children, divide the distance from the navel into six parts. Going down 1 *cùn* from Jiūwěi is the place. Apply moxibustion to both sides at the same time.

(7) Next, apply moxibustion to Wèiguǎn.

(8) Next, apply moxibustion to Jīnmén.[6] Jīnmén is located in front of the grain duct, behind the scrotum, in the very center. Measure the distance from below the scrotum to in front of the anus and divide it in half.

---

1 I read *zhuǎn* 轉 here not literally as "rotating" but in the sense of *zhuǎn jīn* 轉筋, literally "twisted sinews."

2 REN-17 ("Chest Center").

3 In other literature, this is simply used as an alternate name for the preceding point Tánzhōng, but that is obviously not what it means here.

4 REN-8 ("Middle of the Navel").

5 ST-18 ("Hemp Breathing").

6 Metal Gate, 金門 (REN-1). Here, this is an alternate name for the point more commonly known as Huìyīn 會陰 ("Meeting of Yīn," i.e., the perineum) and does not refer to the modern point UB-63.

（一）上腹部十二處，胸堂、巨闕、胃管，十日兒可灸三壯，一月以上可五壯。

（二）陰下縫中可三壯，或云隨年壯。

（一）若脊強反張，灸大椎，並灸諸臟俞，及督脊上當中，從大椎度至窮骨，中屈，更從大椎度之，灸度下頭，是督脊也。

（二）上背部十二處。

（三）十日兒可灸三壯，一月以上可灸五壯。

III.19 Fulminant Seizures

III.19.5

(1) Above, there are twelve locations listed for the abdominal section. On Xiōngtáng, Jùquè, and Wèiguǎn, you can burn three cones on a ten-day-old child, and five cones on a child older than one month.

(2) In the center of the seam below the genitals, you can burn three cones. Alternatively, it is said that you should burn a number of cones that is equal to the patient's years of age.

III.19.6

(1) If [the patient is suffering from] arched-back rigidity, apply moxibustion to Dàzhuī and at the same time to the various *shù* points of the *zàng* organs, as well as to the very center of Dūjí ("Governor Spine"). Measure the distance from Dàzhuī to Qiónggǔ,[1] halve that, and then measure that distance from Dàzhuī down. Apply moxibustion to the bottom end of this measurement. This is Dūjí.

(2) Above, there are twelve locations listed for the section of the back.

(3) On a ten-day-old child, you can burn three cones [on each point]; on a child older than one month, you can burn five cones.

1 DU-1 ("End Bone").

（一）若手足掣瘲，驚者，灸尺澤。

（二）次灸陽明。

（三）次灸少商。

（四）次灸勞宮。

（五）次灸心主。

（六）次灸合谷。

（七）次灸三間。

（八）次灸少陽。

III.19 Fulminant Seizures

III.19.7

(1) If you see tugging and slackening in the hands and feet as well as fright, apply moxibustion to Chǐzé.[1]

(2) Next, apply moxibustion to Yángmíng ("Yáng Brightness").[2]

(3) Next, apply moxibustion to Shàoshāng.[3]

(4) Next, apply moxibustion to Láogōng.

(5) Next, apply moxibustion to Xīnzhǔ.[4]

(6) Next, apply moxibustion to Hégǔ.[5]

(7) Next, apply moxibustion to Sānjiān.[6]

(8) Next, apply moxibustion to Shàoyáng ("Lesser Yáng").[7]

---

1 Now identified with LU-5 ("Cubit Marsh").

2 A rarely used point, described in the *Qiān Jīn Yī Fāng* as located on the back of the big toe, 3 *cùn* from the edge of where the toe separates from the foot ("足拇指奇三寸"). Given the comment in the following line, however, that these points are all located on the hand, it is my best guess that this term refers to a point on the Yángmíng channel that is located on the hand. See below, line III.19.8, for a reference that they are simply located on the fourth digit of the hand and foot, respectively.

3 LU-11 ("Lesser Shāng").

4 PC-7 ("Heart Governor").

5 LI-4 ("Union Valley").

6 LI-3 ("Third Space").

7 A rarely used point, described in the *Qiān Jīn Fāng* as located on top of the second toe, 1 *cùn* behind the first joint. Nevertheless, similar to the point Yángmíng referenced in note 2 above, this must refer to a point on the hand that is used to access the Hand Shàoyáng channel.

（一）上手部十六處。

（二）其要者，陽明、少商、心主、尺澤、合谷、少陽也，壯數如上。

（一）又灸伏兔，次灸三里，次灸腓腸，次灸鹿溪，次灸陽明，次灸少陽，次灸然谷。

（二）上足部十四處，皆要可灸，壯數如上。

（三）手足陽明，謂人四指，凡小兒驚癇皆灸之。

（四）若風病大動，手足掣瘲者，尽灸手足十指端，又灸本節後。

III.19 Fulminant Seizures

III.19.8

(1) Above, there are 16 locations listed for the section of the hand.

(2) Its most important ones are Yángmíng, Shàoshāng, Xīnzhǔ, Chǐzé, Hégǔ, and Shàoyáng. The number of cones [to burn] is the same as above.

III.19.9

(1) Moreover, apply moxibustion to Fútù,[1] next to Sān Lǐ,[2] next to the calf of the leg, next on Lùxī ("Deer Ravine"),[3] next on Yángmíng, next on Shàoyáng, and next to Rángǔ.[4]

(2) Above, there are 14 locations listed for the section of the foot, all of which are crucial and can be treated with moxibustion, with the number of cones calculated like above.

(3) Hand and foot Yángmíng refer to the person's fourth digits. In all cases of fright palpitations in small children, apply moxibustion to all of them.

(4) If [the patient is suffering from] wind disease with severe stirring and tugging and slackening in the hands and feet, apply moxibustion to the ends of every one of the ten digits of the hands and feet. Again, apply moxibustion to the back of the base joints.

1 ST-32 ("Crouching Rabbit").

2 ST-36 ("Three Lǐ").

3 This point name is not attested elsewhere, but based on the progression of points here, it is possible that this refers to Jiěxī 解溪 ("Ravine Divide", ST-41).

4 KI-2 ("Blazing Valley").

Chapter Four: Intrusive Upset
客忤第四

(2 essays, 32 treatments,
1 moxibustion method, 2 spells)

論曰

（一）少小所以有客忤病者，是外人來氣息忤之，一名中人，是為客忤也。

（二）雖是家人或別房異戶，雖是乳母及父母，或從外還，衣服經履鬼神粗惡暴氣，或牛馬之氣，皆為忤也。

（三）執作喘息，乳氣未定者，皆為客忤。

（四）其乳母遇醉或房勞，喘後乳兒最劇，能殺兒也，不可不慎。

IV.1 Essay

IV.1.1 Definition of Intrusive Upset

(1) The reason why the disease of intrusive upset[1] exists in very early childhood is that an outside person has come [into the home] whose qì and breath has caused the upset. Another name is "striking the person." This is what intrusive upset means.

(2) Whether it was a family member or an outsider from another household, whether it was the wet nurse or even the mother or father, perhaps somebody returned from outside and on their clothing or shoes [brought in] the coarse malignancy and fulminant qì of demons and spirits, or it could have been the qì of cattle or horses. All of these [can] cause upset.

(3) Gasping for breath as the result of being grabbed[2] when the breast milk qì has not yet settled[3] [can] always cause intrusive upset.

(4) If the wet nurse has experienced intoxication or taxation from sexual intercourse, is panting,[4] and then breastfeeds the child, this is the gravest [offense] and can kill the child. You must not be careless about this.

---

1 See Commentary IV.1 and Commentary IV.2 on pages 236 and 237.

2 In the *Sūn Zhēn Rén* edition, *zhí* 執 is replaced with *rè* 熱 ("heat"). The entire phrase then becomes: Panting caused by heat and...."

3 *Rǔ qì wèi dìng* 乳氣未定: The meaning of this phrase is slightly obscure, but my best guess is that it refers to the mother or wet nurse feeding the baby when her qì is unsettled, which can certainly affect the baby negatively. See chapter 1, line I.8 on "Selecting a Wet Nurse", p. 47 for some stern warnings about the effect of the wet nurse's emotional state on the baby's health.

4 *Chuǎn* 喘: Literally "panting" or "gasping for breath," this could also be interpreted here as a reference to a wet nurse who is suffering from asthma.

Commentary IV.1 ▻ Sabine Wilms

Kè wǔ 客忤: Wiseman translates this technical term as "visiting hostility." Given the importance and severity of this condition in pediatrics, I would like to reflect the connotations of the Chinese original more literally and strongly. *Kè* 客 clearly has a negative connotation here that is not reflected by the English "guest" or "visiting," the character's more common meaning in modern Chinese. In the classical medical context, however, it can have a strongly negative meaning, similar to the character *zhòng* 中 in the sense of being "struck" by a malign evil force, or qì, invading the body from the outside. The historian of Daoism Catherine Despeux has therefore, in the context of the doctrine of *wǔ yùn liù qì* 五運六氣 ("Five Movements and Six Qì) suggested that we translate *kè qì* 客氣 as "alien qì" (I am grateful to Yi-Li Wu for bringing this elegant solution to my attention.). Regarding *wǔ* 忤, the *Shuō Wén Jiě Zì* glosses it as *nì* 逆 in the sense of "counterflow," "acting against the common or proper direction," or even "rebellion." The most common connotation of *wǔ* is that of being obstinate, insubordinate, refusing to follow orders, or acting against orders, while an alternate meaning is "to touch." The compound *kè wǔ* 客忤 is given in the *Zhū Bìng Yuán Hòu Lùn* as a synonym for *cù wǔ* 卒忤 "sudden upset," which is a subcategory of *zhòng è* 中惡 ("malignancy strike"). There, that compound is explained as caused by a weakness in the person's *jīngshén* 精神 ("essence spirit"), as a result of which the qì of *hún* souls and spirits suddenly strikes it. "Sudden upset" is explained as follows: "Evil intrusive qì suddenly violates and upsets (*fàn wǔ* 犯忤) the person's essence spirit. This is the toxic qì of ghosts and demons and in the category of malignancy strike... Because people have a weakness in their *hún* and *pò* souls, demonic qì intrudes and causes upset. There is a tendency to contract this while on the road outside the home." See the entry on *cù wǔ* 卒忤 in the section on *zhòng è* 中惡 in the *Zhū Bìng Yuán Hòu Lùn*.

Commentary IV.2 ▻ Brenda Hood

Using a more modern understanding, the concept of intrusive upset could be explained by the fact that the protective qì barriers of the newborn are not formed yet and are particularly sensitive to disruption by the qì bodies of others, especially strangers. The character complex used includes the word for guest (*kè* 客) and the word that is here translated as upset (*wǔ* 忤). The character 客 is commonly used in Chinese to indicate something foreign to self or coming from a hostile outside. The character 忤 could also be translated as insubordinate, implying a kind of failing to work within a hierarchy of regulation and hence resulting in upset.

論曰

（一）凡諸乘馬行，得馬汗氣臭，未盥洗易衣裝，而便向兒邊，令兒中馬客忤。

（二）兒卒見馬來，及聞馬鳴驚，及馬上衣物馬氣，皆令小兒中馬客忤，慎護之。特重一歲兒也。

（一）凡小兒衣，布帛綿中不得有頭髮，履中亦爾。

（二）白衣青帶，青衣白帶，皆令中忤。

（三）凡非常人及諸物從外來，亦驚小兒致病。

（四）欲防之法，諸有從外來人及有異物入戶，當將兒避之，勿令見也。

（五）若不避者，燒牛屎，令常有煙氣置戶前則善。

IV.1 Essay

IV.1.2 Horse Intrusive Upset

(1) Whenever people go anywhere on horseback, they come into contact with horses' sweat and stench. If they then, without having washed up and changed their clothes, come to the side of the child, this causes the child to be struck by horse intrusive upset.

(2) If a child suddenly sees a horse coming or hears a horse neighing in panic, [or comes into contact with] the horse qì in the clothes or other things that have been on a horse's back, all of these cause small children to be struck by horse intrusive upset. Beware and protect them against this. This is especially critical in children during the first year of their life.

IV.1.3 Warnings and Taboos for Intrusive Upset in Small Children[1]

(1) Regarding the clothing of small children, the cloth, silk, and padding must never contain any hair from [another person's] head. The same applies to the inside of the shoes.

(2) White clothes with a green-blue belt or green-blue clothes with a white belt all cause [the child] to be struck by upset.

(3) Whenever people or anything else that is out of the ordinary is brought inside from the outside, this also frightens small children and causes this disease.

(4) Here is the method for preventing this: In all sorts of situations where there are people coming in from the outside or strange things entering through the door, ensure that the child avoids them, and do not let them see the child.

(5) If you have failed to avoid them, burn cow dung. Constantly having smoke positioned in front of the door is excellent.

---

1 In the *Sūn Zhēn Rén* edition, this section is preceded by the following heading: *xiǎo ér kè wǔ shèn jì fǎ* 小兒客忤慎忌法 ("Warnings and Taboos for Intrusive Upset in Small Children"). In all other editions, based as they are on the Sòng dynasty revisions by Lín Yì 林億, there is no heading for this paragraph.

論曰

（一）小兒中客為病者，無時不有此病也。

（二）而秋初一切小兒皆病者，豈是一切小兒悉中客邪。

（三）夫小兒所以春冬少病、秋夏多病者，秋夏小兒陽氣在外，血脈嫩弱。

（四）秋初夏末，晨夕時有暴冷，小兒嫩弱，其外則易傷。

（五）暴冷折其陽，陽結則壯熱，胃冷則下痢，是故夏末秋初，小兒多壯熱而下痢也。

（六）未必悉是中客及魃也。

（七）若治少小法，夏末秋初常宜候天氣溫涼也。

（八）有暴寒卒冷者，其少小則多患壯熱而下痢也。

（九）慎不可先下之，皆先殺毒，後下之耳。

IV.1 Essay

IV.1.4 Differentiating Intrusive Upset

(1) If small children fall ill from being struck by intrusion, there are no times when this disease is not present.[1]

(2) And yet, when all the small children at the beginning of autumn without exception fall ill, how could it be that all the small children are comprehensively struck by intrusive evil?

(3) Now the reason why small children suffer fewer illnesses in the spring and winter and more in the fall and summer is that in the fall and summer small children's yáng qì is on the outside and their blood vessels are delicate and weak.

(4) At the onset of autumn and end of summer, if there is fulminant cold at dawn or dusk, since small children are delicate and weak, their outside can easily suffer damage.[2]

(5) Severe cold breaks their yáng, and the yáng binds, resulting in vigorous heat [effusion]. When the stomach gets cold, this results in diarrhea. This is the reason why at the end of summer and beginning of autumn small children often suffer from vigorous heat [effusion] and diarrhea.

(6) This is not necessarily always a case of being struck by intrusion or qí demons.[3]

(7) A rule for treating patients in early childhood: At the end of summer and beginning of autumn, you should constantly watch the weather and temperature.

(8) At times of fulminant cold and sudden cool snaps, very small children will consequently have a tendency to suffer from vigorous heat [effusion] and diarrhea.

(9) Beware! You may not treat this [condition] by moving it downward at first. In all cases, first kill the toxin and then afterwards bring it down!

---

1 Alternatively, this last phrase could possibly be read as "at irregular intervals, they do not have this disease," but the use of 不有 instead of 無 here makes this highly unlikely.

2 The *Sūn Zhēn Rén* edition has *hán* 寒 instead of *bào* 暴 (at the beginning of the next sentence in the current version). This changes the meaning of the phrase to "easily damaged by cold."

3 *Qí* 魃 refers to a type of demon that attacks small children. See chapter three above, Line III.4, note 1, p. 151.

論曰

（一）《玄中記》云：天下有女鳥，名曰姑獲。一名天帝女，一名隱飛鳥，一名夜行游女，又名釣星鬼。

（二）喜以陰雨夜過飛鳴，徘徊人村裡，喚得來者是也。

（三）鳥純雌無雄，不產，陰氣毒化生。

（四）喜落毛羽於人中庭，置兒衣中，便令兒作癎。

（五）病必死，即化為其兒也。

（六）是以小兒生至十歲，衣被不可露也，七八月尤忌。

IV.1 Essay

IV.1.5 Quotation from the *Xuán Zhōng Jì*

(1) A quotation from the *Xuán Zhōng Jì*[1]: "Under heaven, there is a bird-woman called Gū Huò.[2] Another name for her is Tiān Dì Nǚ, another name is Yǐn Fēi Niǎo, another Yè Xíng Yóu Nǚ, another Diào Xīng Guǐ.[3]

(2) On rainy or overcast nights, she likes to fly by, crying out and flying back and forth over the villages of humans. If you call out and you get her to come, this is her.

(3) These birds are pure female, and no males exist. They do not reproduce but are born from transformations of yīn qì poison.

(4) They like to drop their feathers in the courtyards of human dwellings and place them in children's clothing, which then causes the children to suffer from seizures.

(5) This disease invariably ends in death, which means that [the demon] has transformed [the child] to make them her own child.

(6) For this reason, you must not expose the clothes and covers of small children from birth to the age of ten *suì* to the open. Avoid this during the seventh and eighth [lunar] months in particular.

---

1 "Records from the Dark Center," a text by Guō Pú, dating from the Jìn dynasty (265-420).

2 In the *Zhǒu Hòu Fāng*《肘後方》("Treatments to Keep Up One's Sleeve," an important formulary composed during the Jīn dynasty by Gé Hóng) and in the *Zǐ Mǔ Mì Lù*《子母秘錄》("Secret Records for Child and Mother," a now lost text from the Táng dynasty composed by Xǔ Rénzé 許仁則), this bird demon is called Wū Huò 烏獲 ("Black/Crow Catcher"). While Gū Huò could just be a sound, it means, literally translated, "Maiden Catcher." In mythological accounts, she is described as an evil female demon who flies around at night but lies hidden during the daytime. A bird when covered in feathers, but a woman when she drops her feathers, she is childless and therefore loves to steal human children. She does have breasts on her chest. Elsewhere in the *Xuán Zhōng Jì*, she is also described as an evil spirit who likes to seduce people when disguised as a beautiful maiden.

3 Literally translated, these names mean "Heavenly Emperor's Daughter," "Bird Flying in Obscurity," "Night-Roaming Maiden," and "Fisherman's Star Demon," respectively.

論曰

（一）凡中客忤之為病，類皆吐下青黃白色，水穀解離，腹痛夭糾，面色變易，其候似癇，但眼 不上插耳。

（二）其脈急數者是也。

（三）宜與龍膽湯下之，加人參、 當歸，各如龍膽稱分等多少也。

（四）小兒中客，急視其口中懸癰左右。

（五）當有青黑腫脈，核如麻豆大，或赤或白或青，如此便宜用針速刺潰去之。

（六）亦可爪摘決之，並以綿纏釵頭拭去血也。

IV.1 Essay

IV.1.6 Manifestations of Intrusive Upset

(1) All categories of the disease of being struck by intrusive upset manifest with vomiting and diarrhea of a green-blue, yellow, or white substance, separation of water and grain,[1] abdominal pain [to the point of] bending and twisting, and an altered facial complexion, with symptoms that resemble seizures except that the eyes do not roll up towards the ears.

(2) If the pulse is urgent and rapid, this is it.

(3) It is appropriate to give Lóngdǎn Tāng to move [the disease] down, with the addition of *rénshēn* and *dāngguī*, each in an amount equal to the weight of the *lóngdǎn*.

(4) When small children are struck by intrusion, quickly look if there are hanging welling abscesses inside the mouth, on the right or left side.

(5) There will be a green-blue or black swollen vessel with a node the size of a hemp seed, which may be red or white or green-blue. If this is the case, you should use a needle to quickly remove it by piercing and bursting it.

(6) You can also scratch it open with a fingernail. At the same time, wipe away the blood with a hairpin wrapped in silk floss.

---

1 The phrase *shuǐ gǔ jiě lí* 水穀解離 is somewhat unusual, since the more common symptom associated with abdominal upheaval would be its opposite, namely "failure to separate grain and water" (most commonly expressed as 水穀不別), or in other words watery diarrhea with fluids and solids mixed together as the result of incomplete or disordered digestion. Nevertheless, the meaning of the present phrase must be somewhat similar, given the context. One possible interpretation is that solids and fluids are clearly distinguishable in the extreta.

欲療之方

（一）少小中客之為病，吐下青黄赤白汁，腹中痛，及反倒偃側，喘似癇狀。

（二）但目不上插，少睡耳，面變五色，其脈弦急。

（三）若失時不治，小久則難治矣。

（一）用豉數合，水拌令濕，搗熟，丸如雞子大。

（二）以摩兒囟上、手足心各五六遍畢。

（三）以丸摩兒心及臍，上下行轉摩之。

（四）食頃，破視其中，當有細毛，即擲丸道中，痛即止。

IV.2 Treatments For Intrusive Upset

IV.2.1 A Treatment for When You Desire a Cure

Indications

(1) When intrusion strike causes disease in early childhood, it manifests with vomiting and diarrhea of green-blue, yellow, red, or white fluids and pain in the middle of the abdomen, as well as toppling over or bending sideways, and panting that appears like seizures.

(2) Nevertheless, the eyes do not roll upward but the body shakes,[1] the facial complexion changes between the five colors, and the patient's pulse is string-like and urgent.

(3) If you lose the right timing and fail to treat it, such a small condition over a long period of time then becomes difficult to treat!

Preparation

(1) Take several *gě* of *dòuchǐ*, stir it into water to moisten it, and pound it thoroughly. Form a ball about the size of a chicken egg.

(2) Use this to massage the top of the child's skull and the center of the hands and feet, five or six circles each, until you are finished.

(3) Use the ball to massage the child's heart and navel. Massage these areas by going up and down and around in circles.

(4) After the time it takes to eat a meal,[2] break the ball open to see what's in its center. There should be fine hair. Immediately throw the ball into the middle of a road, and the pain will stop right away.

---

1 The *Sūn Zhēn Rén* edition has *mù bù shàng yáo shēn* 目不上，搖身 here instead of 目不上插，少睡耳. Since this is the older version preceding any Sòng editing, I have decided to follow that text in my translation. Punctuating it differently, one could even read this as "the eyes don't shake upward and the complexion of the body and face changes..."

2 I.e., after a little while.

治少小中客忤，強項欲死方：

取衣中白魚十枚，末之，以敷母乳頭上，令兒飲之，入咽立愈。

治少小客忤

竈中黃土、蚯蚓屎等分，擣，合水和如雞子黃大。塗兒頭上及五心良。

IV.2 Treatments For Intrusive Upset

IV.2.2 Another Treatment

Indication
A treatment for being struck by intrusive upset in early childhood, with rigidity in the neck and imminent death:

Preparation
Take ten silverfish,[1] pulverize them, and apply this on top of the mother's nipple. Make the child nurse there so that [the medicine] enters the throat, and recovery will ensue.[2]

IV.2.3 Èr Wù Huángtú Fāng (Two-Ingredient Yellow Dirt Treatment)

Indication
A treatment for intrusive upset in early childhood.

Preparation
Take equal amounts of yellow dirt from inside the stove (*zào zhōng huáng tǔ*) and earthworm excrement. Pound and combine with water until it is about the size of the yolk in a chicken egg. Applying this on top of the child's head and in the five hearts[3] is excellent.[4]

---

1 Literally, "white fish inside clothing," this is an alternate name for a fish-shaped insect that bores its way through clothing or book spines. It is most commonly called *yín* 蟫.

2 Editorial comment: In a variation of this treatment, you use two specimens, placed in the hands of the mother and child and hidden in the child's navel. The child's vomiting and diarrhea mean recovery. Also use [the powdered silverfish] to massage the child's neck and places where the spine is rigid.

3 I.e., the center of the hands and feet and the center of the chest.

4 Editorial comment: A variation calls for mixing it with a chicken's egg white to a mudlike consistency.

又方

（一）吞麝香如大豆許，立愈。

（二）治少小犯客忤，發作有時者方：以母月衣覆兒上，大良。

（三）治小兒卒中忤方：剪取驢前膊胛上旋毛，大如彈子。以乳汁煎之，令毛消。藥成，著乳頭飲之，下喉即愈。

（四）又方：燒母衣帶三寸並發，合乳汁服之。

（五）又方：取牛鼻津服之。

（六）又方：取牛口沫敷乳頭，飲之。

IV.2 Treatments For Intrusive Upset

IV.2.4 Other Treatments

(1) Swallowing an amount of *shèxiāng* about the size of a soybean will cause immediate recovery.

(2) A treatment for attacks of intrusive upset in early childhood, with outbreaks at set times: Cover the child[1] with the mother's menstrual cloth. This is most excellent.

(3) A treatment for small children suddenly struck by upset: Cut off a pellet-sized amount of donkey fur where the animal's hair curls in the front above the shoulder blade. Simmer this in breast milk until the hair is dissolved. When the medicine is ready, apply it to the nipple and have the baby nurse there. When it goes down the throat, recovery ensues.

(4) Another treatment: Burn 3 *cùn* of the mother's cloth belt as well as [an unspecified amount of her] head hair. Combine [the ashes] with breast milk and have the baby ingest it.

(5) Another treatment: Take saliva from a cow's nose and have the baby ingest it.

(6) Another treatment: Take foam from a cow's mouth and rub it onto the nipple. Have the child nurse from there.

---

1 The *Sūn Zhēn Rén* edition has "the child's head."

一物豬蹄散

治小兒寒熱及赤氣中人方：

豬後腳懸蹄，燒末搗篩，以飲乳汁一撮，立效。

治少小卒中客忤，不知人者方：

取熱馬屎一丸，絞取汁飲兒，下便愈。

亦治中客忤而軀啼、面青、腹強者。

IV.2 Treatments For Intrusive Upset

IV.2.5 Yī Wù Zhūtí Sǎn (Single Ingredient Pig's Trotter Powder)

Indication
A treatment for small children suffering from cold and heat as well as from red qì striking the person:

Preparation
Char the dewclaw from a pig's rear leg, then pulverize, pound, and sift it. Give the baby one pinch of this to drink in the breast milk, and recovery will ensue.

IV.2.6 Another Treatment

Indication
A treatment for suddenly being struck by intrusive upset in early childhood, with inability to recognize people:

Preparation
Take one ball of hot horse droppings, wring it out to get the juice, and make the child drink it. A downward movement[1] means that recovery.

It also treats being struck by intrusive upset with bending over and crying, a green-blue face, and a rigid abdomen.

1 I.e., a bowel movement.

二物燒髮散

治少小見人來，卒不佳，腹中作聲者，方：

用向來者人囟上髮十莖，斷兒衣帶少許，合燒灰，細末，和乳飲兒，即愈。

治小兒卒客忤方：

銅鏡鼻燒令紅，著少許酒中，大兒飲之。小兒不能飲者，含與之，即愈。

IV.2 Treatments For Intrusive Upset

IV.2.7 Èr Wù Shāofà Săn (Two-Ingredient Charred Hair Powder)

Indication
A treatment for small children who after being exposed to the arrival of somebody suddenly suffer from unwellness, with sounds in the abdomen:

Preparation
Take ten strands of hair from the top of the head of the person who had arrived and cut off a small length of the child's cloth belt. Combine these and char into ashes, grind them into a fine powder, and mix into breast milk. As soon as you make the child drink this, recovery will ensue.

IV.2.8 Another Treatment

Indication
A treatment for small children who are suddenly suffering from intrusive upset:

Preparation
Heat the nose of a bronze mirror[1] until it is glowing red. Dip it in a small amount of liquor. For larger children, have them drink it. For smaller children who are not able to drink yet, place it in your mouth and give it to them in that way. Recovery will ensue.

1 I.e., the small nob at the back of bronze mirrors where they could be attached to clothing.

一物馬通浴湯

治少小中忤方：

馬通三升，燒令煙絕，以酒一斗煮三沸，去滓，浴兒即愈。

一物豬通浴湯

治小兒中人忤，軀啼、面青，腹強者方。

猳豬通二升，以熱湯灌之，適寒溫浴兒。

IV.2 Treatments For Intrusive Upset

IV.2.9 Yī Wù Mǎtōng[1] Yù Tāng (Single-Ingredient Horse Manure Wash Decoction)

Indication
A treatment for upset strike in early childhood:

Preparation
[Take] 3 *shēng* of horse manure and roast it until the smoking stops. Decoct in 1 *dǒu* of liquor, letting it come to a boil 3 times. Remove the dregs. Bathing the child [in this decoction] causes immediate recovery.

IV.2.10 Yī Wù Zhūtōng Yù Tāng (Single-Ingredient Pig Manure Wash Decoction)

Indication
A treatment for small children who have been struck by human upset, with bending over and crying, a green-blue face, and a rigid abdomen.

Preparation
Take 2 *shēng* of boar manure. Moisten it by pouring hot water over it and bathe the child in it at a comfortable temperature.

1 The *Sūn Zhēn Rén* edition has *mǎ niào* 馬尿 "horse urine" here instead.

《千金要方衍義》

（一）小兒客忤，得之不意間，雖有似乎驚恐，而實未必皆驚。

（二）原其感觸之由，總屬不內外因，略無關乎表裡。

（三）所以治療之法，僅取易辯，不需湯藥。

（四）如衣中白魚，《本經》原治小兒中風項強背起。

（五）麝臍辟邪通經；驢毛截風；牛津通津；豬蹄甲治腹中伏熱。

（六）馬屎汁逐六腑穢毒。馬通浴滌，除血脈諸風。

（七）豬通浴，蒸發胃經邪氣。

（八）竈土、蚓泥，溫中解毒。銅鏡鼻鎮攝肝氣。

（九）已上諸治，總皆取意，以安其心，，所謂醫者意也。

Treatments For Intrusive Upset *Yǎn Yì* (Expanded Meaning)

(1) When small children contract intrusive upset, it happens completely randomly. Even though it can resemble fright and fear, in reality it is not necessarily always [associated with] fright.

(2) The original reason for the contraction always belongs to neither internal nor external causes and is quite unrelated to the exterior or interior [of the patient's body].

(3) Therefore, as far as treatments are concerned, you merely take what is easily differentiated, and do not need to give medicinal decoctions.[1]

(4) Silverfish, for example, are originally described in the *Shén Nóng Běn Cǎo Jīng* as a treatment for wind strike in small children, with a stiff neck that is "riding" on the back.

(5) *Shèxiāng* repels evil and frees the channels. Donkey hair interrupts wind. Cow saliva frees the humors. Pig trotters and hooves treat deep-lying heat inside the abdomen.

(6) The liquid from horse manure expels filth and poison from the six *fǔ* organs, while bathing in horse manure eliminates all kinds of wind from the blood vessels.

(7) Bathing in pig manure effuses evil qì from the stomach channel by steaming it.

(8) Stove ashes and earthworm excrement warm the center and resolve poison. Bronze mirror nose settles and contains liver qì.

(9) The various treatments above generally all have the intention of calming the [patient's] heart. This is what is called the doctor's intention.

1 In other words, you should not look for a deep-lying physical root in the body of the patient, for which complex professional treatment with medicinal substances would be required. The causes for this disease lie outside the patient since the disease strikes at random.

（一）小兒中馬客忤而吐不止者，灸手心主、間使、大都、隱白、三陰交各三壯。

（二）可用粉丸如豉法，並用唾，唾而咒之。

（三）咒法如下。

IV.3 Moxibustion Methods

(1) When small children are struck by horse-type intrusive upset and then vomit incessantly, apply moxibustion to Shǒuxīnzhǔ, Jiānshǐ, Dàdū, Yǐnbái, and Sānyīnjiāo, three cones each.[1]

(2) You can [also] use pills made out of starch as in the method [above] that uses *dòuchǐ*,[2] while at the same time employing spitting. Spit at and pronounce a spell for it.[3]

(3) The spell treatment follows below.

---

1 With the exception of Shǒuxīnzhǔ, these points are generally identified with the modern points PC-5 ("Intermediary Courier"), SP-2 ("Great Metropolis"), SP-1 ("Hidden White"), and SP-6 ("Three-Yīn-Intersection"). Regarding Shǒuxīnzhǔ, no positive identification is possible. The term Shǒuxīnzhǔ ("Hand Heart Ruler") is used in medical literature to refer to the Hand Juéyīn Pericardium channel, but appears to refer to a specific point here. Elsewhere in the *Qiān Jīn Fāng*, Sūn Sīmiǎo does refer to a point named shǒuxīn ("Hand Heart," most likely located right in the center of the palm), as a treatment with moxibustion for ghosts and goblins. So this is most likely identical to the point in this context.

2 This refers to the treatment described in line IV.2.1 on p. 247 above.

3 The object "it" (*zhī* 之) here presumably refers to the pathogenic qì of intrusive upset, whether of equine or human or even demonic origin, or in other words the evil force that is in a way possessing the patient and needs to be exorcised.

咒客忤法

咒曰

摩家公，摩家母，摩家子兒苦客忤。
從我始，扁鵲雖良不如善唾。

良。咒訖，棄丸道中。

IV.4 Spell Treatment For Intrusive Upset

IV.4.1 Spell[1]

Mó jiā gong, mó jiā mǔ, mó jiā zǐ ér kǔ kè wǔ.
Cóng wǒ shǐ, Biǎn Què suī liáng bù rú shàn tuò.

"Massage the father, massage the mother, massage the child who is suffering from intrusive upset.

Since I began, even though Biǎn Què[2] is excellent, he does not reach [my] skill in spitting."

Excellent! When you are finished with the spell, get rid of the pill in the middle of a road.

1 I have intentionally given the *pīnyīn* pronunciation of the spell content here because there is an intrinsic value not only in the meaning but also in the sound of the characters.

2 Biǎn Què was a legendary healer in China's ancient past who was known for his magical ability to diagnose the inner state of the body from no apparent outside signs. He excelled at pulse diagnosis and acupuncture but also at all sorts of other specialties like pediatrics and gynecology, and is sometimes depicted as a bird with a human head.

咒客忤法

又法

（一）取一刀横著竈上，解兒衣，發其心腹訖。

（二）取刀持向兒咒之唾，輒以刀擬向心腹，啡啡曰：

煌煌日，出東方，背陰向陽。
葛公，葛公，不知何公。
子來不視，去不顧，過與生人忤。
梁上塵，天之神；戶下土，鬼所經。
大刀、環、犀，對竈君。

（一）二七唾客愈。

（二）兒驚，唾啡啡如此二七啡啡。

（三）每唾以刀擬之。

（四）咒當三遍乃畢。

（五）用豉丸如上法，五六遍訖。

（六）取此丸破視，其中有毛，棄丸道中，客忤即愈矣。

IV.4 Spell Treatment For Intrusive Upset

IV.4.2 Another Method

Line 1

(1) Take a knife and lay it horizontally on top of the stove. Release the child's clothing and expose his or her heart and abdomen completely.

(2) Now take the knife and hold it toward the child while pronouncing the spell and spitting. Abruptly pretend to [thrust] the knife in the direction of the heart and abdomen. With a *fēifēi* sound,[1] say the following:

Line 2

Huáng huáng rì, chū dōng fang, bèi yīn xiàng yáng.
Gě Gōng, Gě Gōng, bù zhī hé gōng.
Zǐ lái bù shì, qù bù gù, guò yǔ shēng rén wǔ.
Liáng shàng chén, tiān zhī shén; hù xià tǔ, guǐ suǒ jīng.
Dà dāo, huán, xī, duì zào jūn.

"Brilliant sun, emerging from the East, with yīn to the back, facing towards yáng!

Duke Gě, Duke Gě, not knowing Duke What!

You come without looking ahead, leave without turning back, and in passing give living humans [intrusive] upset!

Dust on the roof beam, spirits from Heaven! Dirt under the doorway, passage of ghosts!

Broadsword, ring, rhinoceros horn: directed at the stove god!"

1 This is variously described as the sound made when spitting or vomiting.

咒客忤法

又法

（一）取一刀横著竈上，解兒衣，發其心腹訖。

（二）取刀持向兒咒之唾，輒以刀擬向心腹，啡啡曰：

煌煌日，出東方，背陰向陽。
葛公，葛公，不知何公。
子來不視，去不顧，過與生人忤。
梁上塵，天之神；戶下土，鬼所經。
大刀、環、犀，對竈君。

（一）二七唾客愈。

（二）兒驚，唾啡啡如此二七啡啡。

（三）每唾以刀擬之。

（四）咒當三遍乃畢。

（五）用豉丸如上法，五六遍訖。

（六）取此丸破視，其中有毛，棄丸道中，客忤即愈矣。

IV.4 Spell Treatment For Intrusive Upset

IV.4.2 Another Method

Line 3

(1) Now spit two times seven[2] times, and the intrusion is cured!

(2) For child panic, spit with a *fēifēi* sound, like this, two times seven times, *fēifēi*.

(3) Each time you spit, wield the knife in pretense.

(4) Perform this spell three times, to make it complete.

(5) Apply the *dòuchǐ* pill [to massage the patient] as in the method above, five or six rounds, and then you are done.

(6) Take this pill, break it open and have a look. In its center there will be hair. Get rid of the ball in the middle of a road, and the intrusive upset is immediately cured!

2 I.e., 14.

小兒魃方

論曰

（一）凡小兒所以有魃病者，是婦人懷娠，有惡神導其腹中胎，妒嫉他小兒令病也。

（二）魃者，小鬼也。妊娠婦人不必悉招魃魅，人時有此耳。

（三）魃之為疾，喜微微下痢，寒熱或有去來，毫毛鬢髮，鬡鬡不悅，是其証也。

（四）宜服龍膽湯。

（五）凡婦人先有小兒未能行，而母更有娠，使兒飲此乳，亦作魃。

（六）令兒黃瘦骨立，髮落壯熱，是其証也。

IV.5 Treatments For [Possession By] *Jì* Demons In Small Children

IV.5.1 Essay

(1) In all cases, the reason why small children have *jì* demon disease is that there was a malign spirit during the mother's pregnancy who was led to the fetus in her abdomen. Feeling envy for another person's child [the *jì* demon] caused the small child to fall ill.

(2) *Jì* demons are young ghosts. Not all pregnant women necessarily attract *jì* demons and goblins. People have these from time to time.

(3) The way in which *jì* [demon possession] manifests as a disease is with a tendency to suffer from very slight diarrhea, with cold and heat that possibly come and go intermittently, and with the fine body hair and the hair on the head and temples all becoming coarse, disordered, and unpleasing. These are its symptoms.

(4) It is suitable to give Lóngdǎn Tāng.

(5) In all cases, when a woman has a previous baby who is not yet able to walk, and the mother becomes pregnant again and then lets the child drink this milk, this also causes *jì* [demonic possession].

(6) It causes the child to suffer from yellowing and emaciation down to the bones, hair loss, and vigorous fevers. These are its symptoms.

小兒魃方

治魃方

（一）炙伏翼熟，嚼哺之。

（二）又方：燒伏翼末，飲服之。

（三）又方：以水二升，煮萹蓄、冬瓜各四兩，取浴之。

白蘚皮湯

治少小客魃挾實方

白蘚皮	
大黃	
甘草	（各一兩）
芍藥	
茯苓	
細辛	
桂心	（各十八銖）

上七味，㕮咀，以水二升煮取九合，分三服。

IV.5 Treatments For [Possession By] *Jì* Demons In Small Children

IV.5.2 Treatments for *Jì* Demonic Possession

(1) Dry-roast a bat until done, then chew it and feed it [to the patient].

(2) Another treatment: Roast a bat, pulverize it, and have the patient ingest it in liquid.

(3) Another treatment: Decoct 4 *liǎng* each of *biǎnxù* and *dōngguā* in 2 *shēng* of water and use it to bathe the patient.

IV.5.3 Báixiǎnpí Tāng (Dictamnus Decoction)

Indication

A treatment for intrusion by *jì* demon [disease] complicated by repletion in early childhood.

Ingredients

báixiǎnpí	1 *liǎng*
dàhuáng	1 *liǎng*
gāncǎo	1 *liǎng*
sháoyào	18 *zhū*
fúlíng	18 *zhū*
xìxīn	18 *zhū*
guìxīn	18 *zhū*

Preparation

Pound the seven ingredients above and decoct in 2 *shēng* of water until reduced to 9 *gě*. Divide into three doses.

小兒魃方《千金要方衍義》

（一）魃病，雖云觸魃所致，既病而加乳食不化，結積乳癖，所以腹大寒熱。

（二）龍膽湯一方，專主嬰兒胎熱驚癇，又為魃病首推。

（三）虛加人參、當歸，以助氣血，方可任蜣蜋、大黃之猛。

（四）次則白鮮皮湯，較前風癇方中白羊鮮湯功力稍遜。

（五）白鮮皮專解風毒，故風癇亦多用之。

（六）大黃蕩滌腸胃，有推陳致新之功。

（七）芍藥除堅積腹痛，茯苓治胸脅逆氣，細辛治百節拘攣，桂心利關節結氣，甘草和臟腑寒熱，合諸味主治。

（八）則風癇乳癖，無不兼該，何憚魃氣之不釋乎。

（九）伏翼為禽中之魃，《本經》主寒熱結氣，同氣相攻之用。或炙或燒，無不宜之。

（十）篇蓄為治魃專藥，有利水殺蟲之功。冬瓜利大小腸，有壓丹石之勳。

（十一）魃病之治，總不外乎滌除乳癖也。

Treatments For [Possession By] *Jì* Demons In Small Children
Yǎn Yì (Expanded Meaning)

(1) Even though the text says that *jì* demon disease is caused by contact with a goblin, the disease is then further complicated by a failure to transform breast milk and food, so that they bind and accumulate, causing milk indigestion.[1] For this reason, [the patient suffers from] an enlarged abdomen and from cold and heat.

(2) The formula for Lóngdǎn Tāng is specifically indicated for infants suffering from fetal heat and panic seizures, and it is also the primary [treatment] for *jì* demon disease.

(3) For vacuity, add *rénshēn* and *dāngguī* to assist the qì and blood. This is the only way that [such patients] can tolerate the fierce action of *qiāngláng* and *dàhuáng*.

(4) Next, there is Báixiǎnpí Tāng. Compared with the formula for Báiyángxiān Tāng among the formulas for wind seizures above[2], its effect is slightly more reserved.

(5) *Báixiǎnpí* specifically resolves wind toxin and is therefore also used frequently for wind seizures.

(6) *Dàhuáng* flushes the intestines and stomach clean and has the effect of pushing out the old to make the new to arrive.

---

1 Wiseman translates *rǔ pǐ* 乳癖 as "mammary aggregations," which is indeed an alternative meaning of the term. Nevertheless, the context here makes it clear that the symptom is affecting the baby, not the mother, and is related to digestive problems. I therefore translate *pǐ* 癖 here as indigestion. In the *Guǎng Yùn* 《廣韻》 dictionary from the Sòng period, this character is defined as "abdominal disease" (腹病); in the *Yù Piān* 《玉篇》 dictionary from 543, as "failure to digest food."

2 See pp. 151-153

小兒魃方《千金要方衍義》

（一）魃病，雖云觸魃所致，既病而加乳食不化，結積乳癖，所以腹大寒熱。

（二）龍膽湯一方，專主嬰兒胎熱驚癇，又為魃病首推。

（三）虛加人參、當歸，以助氣血，方可任蜣蜋、大黃之猛。

（四）次則白鮮皮湯，較前風癇方中白羊鮮湯功力稍遜。

（五）白鮮皮專解風毒，故風癇亦多用之。

（六）大黃蕩滌腸胃，有推陳致新之功。

（七）芍藥除堅積腹痛，茯苓治胸脅逆氣，細辛治百節拘攣，桂心利關節結氣，甘草和臟腑寒熱，合諸味主治。

（八）則風癇乳癖，無不兼該，何憚魃氣之不釋乎。

（九）伏翼為禽中之魃，《本經》主寒熱結氣，同氣相攻之用。或炙或燒，無不宜之。

（十）篇蓄為治魃專藥，有利水殺蟲之功。冬瓜利大小腸，有壓丹石之勳。

（十一）魃病之治，總不外乎滌除乳癖也。

Treatments For [Possession By] *Jì* Demons In Small Children *Yǎn Yì* (Expanded Meaning), cont.

(7) *Sháoyào* eliminates solid accumulations and abdominal pain; *fúlíng* treats counterflow qì in the chest and rib-sides; *xìxīn* treats hypertonicity in the hundred joints; *guìxīn* disinhibits the joints and bound qì; and *gāncǎo* harmonizes the viscera and bowels and cold and heat. By combining all these ingredients, [this formula] is the main indication for this treatment.

(8) As a result, with wind seizures and milk indigestion always belonging together, why would you dread not being able to get rid of[3] *jì* demon qì?

(9) The bat is the goblin among the wild animals. According to the *Shén Nóng Běn Cǎo Jīng*, it governs cold and heat and bound qì and has the effect of attacking qì that is identical to its own. Whether you roast or dry-roast it, it is never not suitable.

(10) *Biǎnxù* is the specific medicinal for treating *jì* demons. It has the effect of disinhibiting water and killing bugs. *Dōngguā* benefits the large and small intestines and has the merit of quelling the effects of cinnabar.

(11) The treatment of *jì* demon disease never goes beyond the scope of flushing out and eliminating milk indigestion.

3 *Shì* 釋 literally means to "set free" or "release," but can also mean "to explain."

小兒夜啼方

龍角丸

主小兒五驚夜啼方。

龍角	三銖
牡蠣	九銖，一作牡丹
黃芩	半兩
蚱蟬	二枚
牛黃	如小豆，五枚
川大黃	九銖

（一）上六味，末之，蜜丸如麻子。

（二）蓐裡兒服二丸，隨兒大小，以意增減之。

IV.6 Treatments For Nighttime Crying In Small Children

IV.6.1 Lóngjiǎo Wán (Dragon Horn Pill)

Indication
A formula that governs the five [forms of] panic and nighttime crying in small children.

Ingredients

lóngjiǎo	3 *zhū*
mǔlì	9 *zhū*, a variation of this formula calls for *mǔdān*
huángqín	0.5 *liǎng*
zhàchán	2 pcs
niúhuáng	5 pieces the size of mung beans
dàhuáng	from Sichuan, 9 *zhū*

Preparation
(1) Pulverize the six ingredients above and form into honey pills the size of hemp seeds.

(2) For a baby still in childbed[1], administer two pills [per dose]. Increase or reduce the dosage at your discretion in accordance with the child's size.[2]

1 *Rù lǐ ér* 蓐裡兒: I have purposely translated this phrase somewhat awkwardly to accurately express its specific meaning. It does not refer to a baby in the cradle or simply on a mattress (as the character *rù* can sometimes be interpreted), but in the present context to a newborn baby who is still lying in the straw bedding that was prepared for the mother for childbirth, in order to safely contain all by-products of the birthing process.
2 Editorial comment: Master Cuī 崔氏 calls this formula "Five Frights Pill."

小兒夜啼方

芎藭散

治小兒夜啼，至明即安寐方。

芎藭	
白朮	
防己	各半兩

（一）上三味，治下篩，以乳和，與兒服之，量多少。

（二）又以兒母手掩臍中，亦以摩兒頭及脊，驗。

（三）二十日兒，未能服散者，以乳汁和之，服如麻子一丸。

（四）兒大，能服藥者，以意斟酌之。

IV.6 Treatments For Nighttime Crying In Small Children

IV.6.2 Xiōngqióng Săn (Chuanxiong Powder)

Indication

A treatment for small children's nighttime crying [that is so bad that] they are only able to calm down and fall asleep by dawn.

Ingredients

xiōngqióng	0.5 *liăng*
báizhú	0.5 *liăng*
fángjĭ	0.5 *liăng*

Preparation

(1) Finely pestle[1] and sift the three ingredients above. Mix into breast milk and administer to the child in any amount.

1 *Zhì* 冶: According to Donald Harper, this character should be interpreted as *yě* 冶 in the context of medicinal preparation, which is a metallurgical term that can mean "to hammer metal." Harper therefore renders it as "to smith" in the sense of finely pounding drugs, a labor-intensive technique for processing drugs. "...Sifting techniques were not common in medicine until the Hàn period. Before that time, long pestling was necessary to reduce the drug to a fine powder; and 冶 'smith' was borrowed from metallurgy to denote the pounding process. 冶 appears frequently in *Wŭ wēi* 武威 prescriptions but is rare in later medical literature (and when it does appear in the received literature it is regularly miswritten as 治). Evidently, the word 冶 became obsolete once sifting simplified the process of pulverizing drugs (Early Chinese Medical Literature, p. 223)." In the *Qiān Jīn Fāng*, the character is used consistently for the preparation of powders in the phrase "finely pestle and sift" (*zhì shāi xià* 冶篩下). As the essay on "compounding medicines" (*Hé hé* 合和) in Volume One of the *Qiān Jīn Fāng* states, "When sifting [drugs to prepare] medicinal pills, use heavy and tightly woven thin silk cloth to make it fine, so that they are easily cooked with honey into pills. When sifting [drugs to prepare] medicinal powders, with herbal drugs use light coarse silk, so they will not clump when taken in liquor. With mineral drugs, also use a fine silk sieve to [prepare them] like pill drugs. Whenever you have sifted [the drugs into] a medicinal powder or pill, always mix them again in a mortar, pounding them with a pestle several hundred times. It is best when you can see that the patterns of the colors are all mixed uniformly (Sabine Wilms, unpublished manuscript)."

小兒夜啼方

芎藭散

治小兒夜啼，至明即安寐方。

芎藭	
白朮	
防己	各半兩

（一）上三味，治下篩，以乳和，與兒服之，量多少。

（二）又以兒母手掩臍中，亦以摩兒頭及脊，驗。

（三）二十日兒，未能服散者，以乳汁和之，服如麻子一丸。

（四）兒大，能服藥者，以意斟酌之。

IV.6 Treatments For Nighttime Crying In Small Children

IV.6.2 Xiōngqióng Sǎn (Chuanxiong Powder)

Preparation, cont.

(2) Furthermore, have the child's mother cover [the child's] navel with her hand and also [use this][2] to massage the child's head and spine. Proven to be effective!

(3) For a child within the first twenty days of life, who is not yet able to ingest powders, combine it with breast milk and administer one pill the size of a hemp seed per dose.

(4) For older children who are able to take medicine, use your discretion to dose it attentively.

2 While my translation may strike the reader as a little awkward, the Chinese source does specify that you have to use the mother's hand to massage the child, and I have therefore maintained that meaning in English.

小兒夜啼方

一物前胡丸

（一）治少小夜啼方。

（二）前胡隨多少，擣末，以蜜和丸如大豆。

（三）服一丸，日三。稍加至五六丸，以瘥為度。

IV.6 Treatments For Nighttime Crying In Small Children

IV.6.3 Yī Wù Qiánhú Wán (Single-Ingredient Peucedanum Pill)

Indication
(1) A treatment for nighttime crying in early childhood.

Preparation
(2) Take an appropriate amount of *qiánhú*, pound it into a powder, and combine with honey to form pills the size of soy beans.

(3) Take one pill [per dose], three times a day. Gradually increase it to five or six pills, using [the patient's] recovery as your measure.

小兒夜啼方

（一）又方：以妊娠時食飲偏有所思者物，以此哺兒則愈。

（二）又方：交道中土、伏龍肝各一把。上二味，治下篩，水和少許飲之。

（三）又方：取馬骨燒灰，敷乳上飲兒，啼即止。

（四）治小兒夜啼不已，醫所不治者方：取狼屎中骨，燒作灰末，水服如黍米粒大二枚，即定。

（五）治小兒驚啼方：取雞屎白熬末，以乳服之，佳。

（六）又方：酒服亂髮灰。

（七）又方：臘月縛豬繩，燒灰服之。

（八）又方：燒蝟皮三寸灰，著乳頭飲之。

（九）又方：車轄脂如小豆許，納口中及臍中。

IV.6 Treatments For Nighttime Crying In Small Children

IV.6.4 Unnamed Treatments

(1) Another treatment: Take any substances that [the mother] was craving to eat or drink more than normally when she was pregnant, and feed these to the child. Recovery will ensue.

(2) Another treatment: Take one handful each of dirt from the middle of a crossroads and *fúlónggān*.[1] Finely pestle and sift the two ingredients above and combine with water. Drink it by sipping a little at a time.

(3) Another treatment: Take horse bones and char into ashes. Spread this on the [mother's] breast and have the child nurse. The crying will stop immediately.

(4) A treatment for small children's incessant nighttime crying, which has not responded to medical treatment: Remove bones from wolf droppings. Char into ashes and pulverize. Take two pieces the size of millet grains and swallow with water. This will settle it.

(5) A treatment for panic [and] crying in small children: Take *jīshǐbái* (i.e., the white in chicken droppings), simmer and pulverize it. Administer this in breast milk. Excellent!

(6) Another treatment: Char *luànfà* (disheveled hair) into ashes and administer in liquor.

(7) Another treatment: Char a rope that was used to tie up a pig in the twelfth month into ashes and administer that.

(8) Another treatment: Char a 3-*cùn* [piece] of *wèipí* (hedgehog skin) into ashes, apply to the [mother's] nipple, and have [the child] nurse from there.

(9) Another treatment: Place a mung bean-sized piece of cart axle grease into the [child's] mouth and in the middle of the navel.

---

1 Alternate name for *zàoxīntǔ*.

小兒夜啼方

千金湯

主小兒暴驚啼絕死，或有人從外來，邪氣所逐，令兒得疾，眾醫不治方：

蜀椒	
左顧牡蠣	各六銖，碎

上二味，以醋漿水一升，煮取五合，一服一合。

IV.6 Treatments For Nighttime Crying In Small Children

IV.6.5 Qiān Jīn Tāng (Thousand Gold Decoction)

Indication

A treatment indicated for small children suffering from fulminant panic and crying to the point of expiry or death. Maybe a person came in from the outside who was followed by evil qì, and this caused the child to contract the illness. [For cases that] multitudes of physicians have failed to treat:

Ingredients

shǔjiāo	6 *zhū*, smashed
left-facing *mǔlì*	6 *zhū*, smashed

Preparation

Decoct the two ingredients above in 1 *shēng* of fermented millet drink[1] until reduced to 5 *gě*. Take 1 *gě* per dose.

1 This is the literal translation of this term, which is also used elsewhere in the *Bèi Jí Qiān Jīn Yào Fāng*, but not attested in other received medical literature. According to the *Běn Cǎo Gāng Mù* (vol. 5), *jiāng* 漿 alone refers to a fermented alcoholic beverage, made by soaking heated millet in water for five or six days. It is most often called *jiāng shuǐ* 漿水

小兒夜啼方《千金要方衍義》

（一）方書論小兒夜啼，但以見火而啼為胎熱，去火而啼為胎寒。

（二）此辨固是，但未及胎風胎驚，胸腹脹痛等，治不若《千金》之兼到也。

（三）如龍角丸專取東方木氣，以透肝風。

（四）牡蠣以斂腎氣，大黃以滌驚痰，黃芩以解風熱，牛黃以定胎驚，蚱蟬專止夜啼，為胎熱驚啼峻藥。

（五）芎藭散專取芎藭以散風熱，白朮以培土虛，防己以開痰癖，為滌熱安中專藥。

（六）前胡丸但取一物以下痰氣，為表虛胎風善藥。

（七）千金湯專取川椒以溫中氣，牡蠣以鎮腎怯，為腎虛胎寒要藥。

Treatments For Nighttime Crying In Small Children *Yǎn Yì* (Expanded Meaning)

(1) The formulary literature discusses the issue of nighttime crying in early childhood, but merely notes that if the baby cries when seeing fire this means fetal heat (*tāi rè* 胎熱) and if the baby cries when you remove the fire this means fetal cold (*tāi hán* 胎寒).

(2) This differentiation is certainly solid, but it fails to take into account such aspects of fetal wind, fetal panic, distention and pain in the chest and abdomen, etc. The treatments [listed in the other formula texts] therefore do not compare with the treatments in the *Qiān Jīn Fāng*.

(3) For example, Lóngjiǎo Wán specifically utilizes wood qì from the eastern direction, in order to outthrust liver wind.

(4) *Mǔlì* is used to restrain kidney qì; *dàhuáng* to sweep away panic phlegm; *huángqín* to resolve wind heat; and *niúhuáng* to settle fetal panic; while *zhàchán* specifically stops nighttime crying. This is a drastic medicine for fetal heat-related panic and crying.

(5) Xiōngqióng Sǎn specifically uses *xiōngqióng* to scatter wind heat; *báizhú* to shore up earth vacuity; and *fángjǐ* to open phlegm aggregations. It is a medicine specifically for sweeping away heat and quieting the center.

(6) Qiánhú Wán merely utilizes a single ingredient to bring down phlegm qì. It is an excellent medicine for exterior vacuity and fetal wind.

(7) Qiān Jīn Tāng specifically utilizes *chuānjiāo* to warm center qì and *mǔlì* to settle kidney timidity. It is an essential medicine for kidney vacuity and fetal cold.

小兒夜啼方《千金要方衍義》

（一）伏龍肝以填土虛，交道土以通脾氣，為脾虛胎熱良藥。

（二）其馬骨灰、狼屎骨皆主胎風。猬皮灰除胃脘痛。雞矢白治腹脹滿。

（三）亂髮灰專主胎驚，隨證取用血肉之味也。

（四）設治都不應，則以其母懷身時所思之物哺兒，以適胎情，為不藥之藥。

（五）曲盡夜啼治法矣。

Treatments For Nighttime Crying In Small Children *Yǎn Yì* (Expanded Meaning), cont.

(1) *Fúlónggān* is used to shore up earth vacuity, and crossroads dirt to free the flow of spleen qì. This is an excellent medicine for spleen vacuity and fetal heat.

(2) Both horse bone ashes and the bones in wolf droppings rule fetal wind. Charred hedgehog skin eliminates pain in the stomach and stomach duct. *Jīshǐbái* treats abdominal distention and fullness.

(3) Ashes of *luànfà* specifically rules fetal panic. Thus this is a way of using a flesh-and-blood ingredient in accordance with the pattern.

(4) If [the condition] fails to respond to any of the treatments you have designed, take any of the substances that the mother was craving during pregnancy and feed these to the child, in order to suit the fetus' sentiment. This constitutes a medicine that is not a medicine.

(5) These are the detailed ins and outs of the treatments for nighttime crying.

Weights and Measures

Weights

1 *shǔ* 黍	=	millet grain
1 *zhū* 銖	=	10 *shǔ* 黍
1 *fēn* 分	=	6 *zhū* 銖
1 *liǎng* 兩	=	24 *zhū* 銖
1 *jīn* 斤	=	16 *liǎng* 兩

Volume

1 *dāo guī* 刀圭	=	4 *wútóng* 梧桐
1 *cuō* 撮	=	4 *dāo guī* 刀圭
1 *sháo* 勺	=	10 *cuō* 撮
1 *gě* 合	=	2 *sháo* 勺
1 *shéng* 升	=	10 *gě* 合
1 *dǒu* 斗	=	10 *shéng* 升
1 *hú* 斛		10 *dǒu* 斗

Length

1 *fēn* 分		
1 *cùn* 寸	=	10 *fēn* 分
1 *chǐ* 尺	=	10 *cùn* 寸
1 *bù* 步	=	5 *chǐ* 尺
1 *lǐ* 里	=	1800 *chǐ* 尺

Single Herb & Formula Index

G

H

J

L

M

N

P

Q

R

S

T

U

W

X

Y

Z

Indications Index

V

W

Y

Acupuncture & Moxibustion Index

Points by Channel and Number

Other Points

Channels

Proper Name Index

General Index

G

H

S

www.ingramcontent.com/pod-product-compliance
Lightning Source LLC
Chambersburg PA
CBHW061620220326
41598CB00026BA/3821